The Work in Between

A Memoir About Stepping Out of My Shadows

Gretchen Norling Holmes, PhD

PAGE & PODIUM
PRESS

Foreword

I first met Gretchen when she reached out to me for transformational coaching. She had come across something I had posted and was called to connect. Upon meeting and subsequently working together, her objective was to get "unstuck," not only professionally, but personally. Gretchen was dealing with a significant amount of grief and anger.

She yearned to move forward.

To preface, as a transformational coach, I co-think with my clients. My belief is that my clients are not broken and, therefore, do not need to be fixed. They are complete and whole individuals. I provide a sacred space in which to do the internal work. Gretchen's body had indeed been healed. Now it was time to heal from the inside.

Gretchen's story is one of Strength. Resiliency. And Love.

I would offer that most of us would like to sidestep struggle. Dodge cancer. Skip grief. Gretchen was no different.

The Work in Between depicts the power of love. To love oneself and all around you. Moving beyond cancer survivor to cancer thriver, Gretchen brings forth thoughts of how to navigate the unexpected, the unwanted, and the unknown for the betterment of your own growth.

Gretchen generously shares her own journey of letting go and stepping in. Holding both. Releasing and reaching. Letting go of habits and thought patterns that no longer serve. Reaching for structure that supports. Letting go of perfection. Reaching for self-acceptance and the celebration of each win. Letting go of anger. Reaching and moving forward with love.

I have witnessed Gretchen slowly and intentionally thread the smaller versions of herself and her life experiences to bring forth the biggest version of herself. She has broken through her own limiting thoughts to take control of her life. She is now the architect of her own happiness.

Gretchen's book is about Light. The Light within herself and the Light she brings and shares with the world. Discovering who she is.

We are all seeking to find our health, our grounding, and be in our strength. Be in our own Light. This striving is Universal. We are interconnected.

In this important and timely book, Gretchen Holmes brings forth this Oneness.

The Work in Between offers a look into empowerment, growth, healing, and ultimately, personal transformation through self-love. Through the shares of her own journey as a three-time cancer survivor, succeeding in life-changing weight loss after being diagnosed with diabetes, and processing the loss of her birth family, Gretchen boldly and rawly shares her story, and the layers of her soul's healing.

It is a brave step to share such an important journey of her life —the journey we should all embark upon—learning to love ourselves.

Savor each word and all the thoughts to come.

Marcie Montgomery, CPCC, PCC

Chapter One

In the fall of 1992, during my final year at NYU, I noticed a lump at the base of my throat. It was quite large. About six months before I left for NYU, I remembered a coworker had mentioned that I should consider going to the doctor for my thyroid. She must have noticed the lump there, but I hadn't seen it. I sure noticed it now. I was having trouble swallowing and was sleeping more than usual. Plus, I was rapidly gaining back weight that I had worked hard to lose. I went to student health to see if they could figure out what was going on with me.

The provider did a brief exam of the tumor at the base of my neck.

"I'm not sure what's going on," he said, "but my guess is a goiter. Try adding more salt to your diet. Eat a few of those big New York pretzels." That's ridiculous, I thought. I felt dismissed and disrespected, like he didn't take my situation seriously. I wondered if it was because of my weight.

My gut said there was something else going on with my body, so I had to keep searching for an answer. I went to a physician recommended by a friend. I was in the waiting room when she came through the door with her bicycle. That, in and of itself, wasn't unusual in New York, but it struck me as strange. She also wore a funny hat. I told her that I was having difficulty swallowing. I was gaining a lot of weight. Sleeping more than ever before. My hair was falling out, and my joints were hurting.

She ordered an ultrasound.

"Yep, you have something there, alright," she told me in the follow-up visit. "But I'm a doctor, and it's my job to determine if you're sick or not, and you're not. We can watch it for six months and see what happens."

I was shocked. Frankly, I was speechless. Even I could see the tumor on the ultrasound. It was huge! I was having a harder and harder time swallowing, I was still piling on weight, and I was exhausted. I was getting scared. Going to school full-time, working part-time, and dealing with being sick was too much. I had to find out what was going on.

Although it took longer than I wanted it to, I finally got in to see a third physician that another friend recommended. He was considered one of the top endocrinologists in New York and specialized in thyroid cancer. At least three months had passed since I first noticed the tumor. I was getting beyond impatient.

Upon examination, he decided to immediately perform a fine-needle biopsy. He was concerned that it could be cancer. He gave me no time to prepare myself; he just left the room and brought back in the longest needle I had ever seen. It looked at least six inches long. He used an ultrasound wand to locate the tumor and then he said, "I'm going to inject this needle into your neck. Whatever you do, don't swallow while it's in there."

Have you ever tried to *not* swallow when someone told you not to?

How about when they were sticking a huge needle into your neck?

It was at that moment that I knew it was serious. My instincts are pretty accurate, and I just knew. I slowed my breathing and closed my eyes. He stuck the needle in my neck; I didn't swallow. I didn't move. I barely breathed.

He sent the sample off for evaluation. It was inconclusive, but he recommended surgery anyway. By then, it was clearly necessary because I could hardly swallow and was on a practically liquid diet. Plus, it was becoming more difficult to breathe. I was miserable. I was finding it harder and harder to focus on school, I was exhausted all the time, and I hurt. The tumor had to be removed.

I was due to graduate at the end of the spring term. Missing classes just wasn't an option for me, so I scheduled my surgery during spring break. I knew I wouldn't have enough time to heal before I had to go back to school, but I was too close to realizing my dream. Even though I'm sure my professors would have understood, I wasn't taking that chance. I had my surgery a week later. The doctor thought we might learn more once they opened me up, but during the surgery, they still couldn't figure it out. Once I woke up, I was told that the surgery took longer than expected because they couldn't decide whether they should take both lobes of my thyroid. They had argued about it. Ultimately, they decided to do a partial thyroidectomy and left the other lobe intact. They removed a sample of the tumor, and it was sent to the pathology lab at Sloan Kettering for a "slow grow."

A week later, they removed the drain from my neck. I was back at school the next day. I had to wear a bandage to cover my incision because they hadn't yet taken out my stitches. It was way too soon, but I returned to school anyway.

As I would find out, there's a lot of waiting with thyroid cancer.

Six weeks later, late in the evening, I finally got the call.

"Ms. Norling, it came back cancer. My nurse will call you tomorrow to make a follow-up appointment. I'm sorry."

Cancer. I had cancer.

I just sat there, stunned. My brain shut down. I couldn't breathe. I didn't know what to do. I left work early. A colleague joined me when I stepped into the elevator. I must have had tears in my eyes because he asked me if I was alright.

"I have cancer," I told him.

"Oh. I'm sorry," he said. I didn't know what else to say and I doubt he did, either. We rode the elevator in silence the rest of the way.

Afterward, I kept saying the word cancer out loud. Maybe I thought it would have less power over me. I'm not sure. Magical thinking, I suppose. I told everyone about it. I would slip it into conversations where it didn't belong. I did some of my own research, and I realized that if you're going to have cancer, it was a very treatable cancer to have.

I had thyroid cancer, technically a papillary-follicular variant of thyroid cancer. As I would be told hundreds of times, "If you're going to get cancer, thyroid cancer is the one to get."

I was grateful that it wasn't a more aggressive cancer, but it didn't make it any less stressful or difficult to process.

I followed up with my endocrinologist following the surgery. We talked about Radioactive Iodine Treatment (RAI) which was the normal standard of care.

I had recently gotten married, and we thought maybe we wanted to have children. It seemed risky to do it right then.

＊

I met my first husband in New York at a Chinese restaurant on the Upper West Side. We became friends and as was my pattern, I made an impulsive decision, and we eloped. I called my mom afterward.

"Guess what? I got married!" I could almost hear crickets in the silence that followed.

Finally, she said in a quiet, hurt voice, "I didn't know you were seeing anyone."

I hate that I hurt her that way. Of course, she would want to be a part of my wedding, and I took that away from her. It was one example of a terrible habit of mine that would take years to learn how to break: I made decisions and let the people who would be most affected find out later. I am not proud of that to this day.

A few months later we went to Midland and Mom and Dad threw us a lovely reception. That helped heal the hurt. A little.

I expressed my concerns about RAI to my doctor, but he didn't press the importance of the treatment on me and told me I could wait. Honestly, I couldn't get a straight answer from anyone, my endocrinologist, or my surgeon. As the patient, I ultimately had to make the decision, but without clear communication about my options, it was difficult to make an informed decision. It's incredibly frustrating.

Overall, my encounters with doctors have never been particularly productive. During one office visit with the doctor who had diagnosed my thyroid cancer, I got upset and started to cry, which was highly unusual for me. I had decisions to make, but I was scared and wasn't sure what to do. I didn't understand everything that was happening. I sat there on the exam table with tears rolling down my face, overwhelmed.

He looked at me and said, "I can't help you with that." With that, he walked out of the room.

I felt ashamed that I even brought it up. I was embarrassed and humiliated. Being rejected when I showed vulnerability, especially during a medical visit, destroyed me. It was a huge error in judgment on his part, but that didn't matter in the moment. It completely destroyed any trust or faith I had in him or physicians in general. But

I'm a survivor, and I knew it would be up to me to find my way through this. I dried my tears and got dressed. I met him in his office afterward, as was the routine. There, he showed me pictures of his grandkids and was quite chatty, as though nothing had even happened.

I don't think the cancer registered as much as it would have had I not been so busy and focused on graduating that year. It had taken me a long time to find my rhythm in college, and nothing was going to stop me now that I could see the finish line.

There were papers to write, tests to take. I had to coordinate my family's trip for graduation. And all the while, I had to navigate having cancer. Whichever thing was the most emergent, that's where my attention went. Sometimes it was school, sometimes it was cancer. I couldn't afford to get derailed, so I just kept putting one foot in front of the other. There were so many things competing for my attention that I couldn't just focus on how bad I felt or how nervous I was about having cancer.

Many decades later, when I was in my sixties, I realized that chaos had always been my norm. A chaotic environment wasn't uncomfortable nor foreign to me, which is why I'm not surprised that I did so well during this time in my life and weathered the years of struggles yet to come. Frankly, it was my comfort zone.

I come from a home with heaps of dysfunction and an alcoholic father. Anyone who has experienced addiction in their homes growing up understands the craziness that goes on and how it affects the adults we become. We all have war stories. The names may change, and the intensity varies, but it's a familiar tale to those who have been through it. Adding insult to injury, I was also obese, often morbidly obese, throughout my life until I was diagnosed with diabetes. That would change everything.

I've also had more than my share of blessings. I've met some of the most amazing people, had some of the grandest experiences, and loved so deeply—and been so deeply loved—that it almost seems unfair. Maybe that's part of the reason why I still look forward to the future instead of being pessimistic.

When it came down to it, it wasn't the chaos or the cancer that crippled me. Not that first diagnosis, nor the second, nor the third. It wasn't diabetes or morbid obesity.

Bad things happen to all of us, but it seems some of us get more than our fair share of challenges. I don't know why. I've never been prone to asking, "Why me?" Frankly, my response has pretty much always been, "Why not me?"

This isn't because I felt I deserved it, mind you, it was just because I never thought I was any more or less deserving of good or bad things than anyone else. Sometimes, things just happen. So, in a weird way, I never thought any of it was personal. Maybe that's why I approached my life a little differently.

Growing up, my mom always told me two things:

Bad things happen to everyone. You don't have to build a mountain to them.

Don't compare your insides to other people's outsides.

These adages helped me not to crumble when the world got to be too much. How not to fall victim to events out of my control. As for comparing my insides to other people's outsides? Well, that one was a little harder. I'm still a work in progress, but I think Mom would be proud of the woman I have become.

Actually, I think she would have been proud anyway.

None of those bad things were my biggest obstacle. What paralyzed me were times when I kept secrets.

I couldn't carry all the difficult, confusing, sometimes awful, usually embarrassing things that happened in my life on my own. It was too much to carry. It would eat me up inside and make me physically sick to my stomach. So, over time, I learned to talk about it.

I talked about it with old friends and sometimes even new friends and almost always my teachers. It helped me process it, and it made me feel better. It allowed me to keep moving forward and not become paralyzed with fear and uncertainty. Looking back, I think it ended up being my lifesaver. For me, it normalized talking about subjects that many other people kept in the shadows. Admittedly, I didn't understand the effect that sharing my experiences would have on my life, but what I did know was that I couldn't carry all the trauma on my own. I don't believe anyone can. In retrospect, bringing it into the open lessened the power it had over me.

Chapter Two

Growing up in an alcoholic home was hard. It had a huge impact on my development, of course, because so many of our beliefs about ourselves are established as young children. Trying to make sense of my environment through my young eyes was bound to have a negative impact on my sense of self and it did. As an adult, I realized I was constantly searching for attention and acceptance, which led me to make some unhealthy choices. I was also seeking approval, especially from my dad, and that, too, drove some poor decisions.

But I refuse to blame my childhood for every poor decision, every bad experience, or every problem I've had as an adult. We all have baggage. All of us. At some point, I had to own my agency in my life, especially as I became aware of my role in it. If I refused to consider that it was my actions, thoughts, or beliefs that got me here, I would stay exactly where I was. Stuck. Sick. A victim. My environment may explain why I didn't have the awareness or the tools as a young girl, but as I grew into adulthood, I had choices. We always have choices, but first, I had to become aware of them.

Then, I had to be willing to own what was mine to heal, grow, and prosper.

I grew up in Midland, Michigan in a lower-middle-class family. I was the middle child with an older brother, Chris, and a younger brother, Eric. Dad and Mom both worked; Dad at the chemical plant and Mom at the local newspaper for most of her career. Dad was an active alcoholic for most of my growing-up years, so our lives tended to be chaotic and uncertain—but there was always love. Lots of love. Even with the addiction and the dysfunction, I knew I was deeply loved and so were my brothers.

I also knew our family was different from my friends'. Our lights were periodically turned off for nonpayment and sometimes we left to go stay with my grandma and aunt until Dad went back into treatment. We had lots of good times, though. There was always music and food and extended family around for holidays, birthdays, and weekend picnics. I had tons of aunts, uncles, and cousins, and I loved being with them. They made me laugh and helped me forget my troubles. It wasn't an idyllic childhood, but honestly, who has one of those? Everyone has something to deal with growing up, this just happened to be my thing.

Dad's alcoholism existed for as long as I can remember. He was always drinking too much at parties, when we went camping, and especially on payday. Sometimes, we wouldn't see him for a week after he got paid. His standard line before he went off on a bender was simply: "I'm going out for cigarettes." That's when we knew that he was going to start drinking—maybe just for a day, but it was often for a week or even longer. It was always calmer when he was gone, and I'd feel guilty for thinking that. I loved my dad. I was Daddy's girl from the beginning. But when he was gone, there was no stress, no chaos. Mom was more relaxed. We all were, and even though we usually didn't have enough money, we were a lot happier. We laughed more and slept better.

On the other hand, I worried. All the while he'd be gone, I'd worry about whether he was okay or if he was going to come home drunk or even come home at all. I remember as a very young girl, maybe five or six, beginning to notice an uncomfortable feeling in the pit of my stomach. Not all the time, but it would come up. Mom called them "the dreads." The dreads grew the longer Dad was gone. Coming home on the school bus, I'd look out the window to see if his truck was home, holding my breath. If it wasn't, I'd exhale. If it was, I'd feel the dreads full-on because I wouldn't know what I would be walking into. Was he sober and in a good mood or was he drunk and belligerent? The dreads stayed with me for most of my life.

They still show up from time to time.

Sooner or later, he'd come home, and the chaos would start again. When he was drinking, it wasn't unusual for my dad to come home in the middle of the night after the bars closed. Unfortunately, it was usually during the week, and Mom would have to get up and fix him and his new friends he met at the bar something to eat. At three o'clock in the morning, when Mom had to get up in a few hours to go to work and we had school, there would be a loud party going on in our house. My bedroom was off the dining room and our piano backed up to one of my bedroom walls. Sure enough, when they were done eating, Mom would have to play the piano, which meant no one slept. Mom hated doing all of it, but Dad could become nasty and belligerent, so it was just easier to comply. He was never physically aggressive towards Mom, but I always felt the threat was there. The arguments would come the next day.

The stress was palpable at our house. There was a lot of uncertainty. It wasn't unusual to have our power turned off. Dad was terrible with money, but he always had big dreams, so when he was sober, he would buy things or start some new project that he hadn't really thought through. I found myself doing the exact same thing as an adult.

One day, I came home from school, and he had bought a registered quarter horse for me. I don't know why he thought I wanted a horse. I guess I had mentioned in passing that a friend of mine had one, but I wasn't a horse person. I suppose he was trying to connect with me or be a good dad.

A few weeks later, the horse bit me so he sold it. He didn't ask me if I wanted him to sell it—I just came home one day, and it was gone. We finally figured out years later that the things he bought weren't really for us, even though he said they were, so getting rid of things wasn't really about us either. I'm guessing he sold it to make a house payment so we wouldn't lose our house, or he used it to buy something else or to go out drinking. Who knows. After he sold the horse, he opened a dog food store in our garage. As a young teenager, I ended up manning the store and loading fifty-pound bags of dog food into customer's trucks. I didn't mind doing it, but looking back, it was a lot of responsibility for a thirteen-year-old.

Periodically, Mom would decide to leave. She felt terribly guilty as she got older that she hadn't gotten us out of the situation earlier. Eric and I would try so hard to convince her that she really did do the best she could, but I'm not sure we ever lessened that guilt for her. I wish we could have. We would pack up, occasionally in the middle of the night, and go to Grandma's house. Sometimes, we would even find a new place to live. Most of the time, when Mom would leave, Dad would go to rehab. He loved Mom deeply. He loved us, too, but Mom? He *loved* her. If somehow his alcoholism and his behaviors were separated from how much he truly loved her, it would have been a great love story. Unfortunately, it wasn't. It was all tied together in one messy situation. No matter how much he loved her, he caused a lot of damage. That was why he carried an unbearable amount of guilt once he got sober. Even with everything that happened, I never thought he deserved to carry that level of guilt. No one can survive the amount of guilt my dad had. It haunted him. He rarely talked about it because he couldn't, and we didn't bring it up because we were all so broken.

Guilt is a debilitating emotion, and we all had plenty to go around, along with enough regret to last a lifetime. I wish our family had gone to counseling. We tried here and there, but it wasn't consistent or effective. There was so much to unpack that I'm not sure anyone could have figured it all out.

The dreads would grow as the uncertainty and the craziness increased. The older I got, the more I tried to make sense of a situation no one could make sense of. Strangely, I never felt in danger. How I knew Mom and Dad would never let anyone physically hurt me, I'm not sure, but the situation was taking a terrible emotional toll on all of us. At times, especially as I became a teenager, I rarely came out of my room. It was easier just to avoid whatever was going on.

Throughout my childhood and throughout most of my adult life, I self-soothed with food. I ate when I was sad, happy, scared, bored, or stressed. Whatever the emotion, I ate in response.

Like most children, I didn't have a lot of control at home. I ate what my parents put in front of me. At least, that's how it was at our house. Back then, it wasn't an option to request something else. I didn't know any house where they prepared something different for anyone, especially a kid. You just ate what was served or you didn't eat. At our house, it was meat and potatoes. Comfort food. We usually had a garden so there were vegetables, but that's not what I liked to eat. I liked carbs. My favorite was macaroni and cheese from a box. It still is. To be honest, I wouldn't have asked for anything different anyway. Food was comfort to me, and comfort food was what I craved. It made me feel better. It quieted my anxiety and the questions that would play on repeat in my mind: *When was Dad going to come home? Would he be drunk or sober? If he came home, would there be more arguments? Would I end up in tears? Would I feel scared?*

Food comforted me. It became my best friend.

I have been obese or morbidly obese for most of my life. It's not a reflection on my intelligence nor my character; it's just a fact, not a flaw. It shouldn't have defined me, but it did, just as it defines tens of millions of others who are physically different from everyone else. Being five foot ten, I could carry some extra weight, but it was obvious, of course, as physical issues are. You can't hide it. Wearing black or vertical stripes doesn't cover it up. Unlike some other health issues, being overweight is evident to everyone at all times. We live in an image and beauty-conscious world and for many, being fat is the worst thing you could possibly be! It somewhat explains the fat bias and why it's socially acceptable to shame and berate people who dare to be fat, but it's not the entire explanation. When I discovered online sites dedicated to shaming fat people, it didn't surprise me. Fat shaming is a global problem. Even physicians and nurses who dedicate their lives to working with obesity can carry significant fat bias toward their patients. Trying to live your life in an environment where people go out of their way to make you question your worth or whether you should even exist is unhealthy. It's toxic, but that's what many of us navigate daily. Sometimes that hatred and toxicity come from within; it's exhausting to keep rejecting those negative messages all the time. Sometimes it starts in your home, coming from "well-meaning" parents or relatives, but it's the culture we live in after we leave our homes, too. Often there's no way to escape it inside or out. Something clearly isn't working here. We have a lot of work to do.

As a child, I was aware that I was bigger than other kids my age, but I couldn't do anything about it. I didn't have the ability or resources. As an adult, I tried periodically to lose weight, but I never identified or addressed the underlying issues, beyond just limiting calories. I didn't know what to do. Anyone can lose weight by restricting calories long enough, but considering I wasn't particularly happy when I was doing that, it didn't last long.

Clarity doesn't always come when you want it, neither does wisdom. Also, sometimes, you're so deep into your dysfunction that uncertainty and indecision can be paralyzing. Most times, I couldn't see clearly enough to know what a healthy first step would even be. Frankly, overeating was serving a purpose for me, so I just kept doing it. It made me feel safe, albeit guilty. I knew I was eating too much because I would often sneak food, but it reduced my anxiety, dried my tears, and helped me deal with my emotions. I couldn't stay scared, sad, or worried all the time. No one can. So, I ate.

Chapter Three

If it sounds like life was nothing but misery and chaos, that's not how it was. We lived in a farmhouse out in the country with a large front porch and a big yard with huge, mature shade trees. We spent a lot of time sitting on that front porch talking. Sometimes we were laughing, sometimes we were crying, but in the summer, there was no better place to be than on that front porch. There was always a slight wind blowing which made some of the hot and humid Michigan summers more bearable.

Our family went on long camping trips for vacation in the summer. We had cookouts on the weekends at Grandma's house where there was softball, laughter, lots of good food, and music. Grandma LaMott made every one of us feel like we were the most special person in the world. There was lots of love, and we all felt it. I loved my family deeply. I still do. Even Dad, especially Dad. Even when he was at his worst, when alcoholism and addictions were winning. I still loved him. I hated what he was doing, and what the disease was doing to him, but I loved the man. It wasn't always easy, but he deserved love even when he was making it hard to love him. We all do.

We knew Dad loved us, too. He just had a much harder time showing it. That's not unusual when someone has alcoholism along with emotional and mental issues. His father was also an alcoholic and ultimately died from it. His childhood wasn't a bed of roses, either. What I experienced growing up is not unusual when there's addiction running in the family. It's just not. For those of you who grew up in an alcoholic home (or with any other addiction), I suspect you can relate.

My two brothers and I were very close. Mom used to call us the Norling Mafia. If you messed with one of us, you got all of us. Chris was nearly two years older than me, and Eric was six years younger.

They were extremely talented musicians. Chris played guitar and a few other instruments, but he played the mandolin unlike anyone we'd ever heard. Eric played the bass. Together, they had a band called the Seventh Street Band. Chris especially became well-known for his musicianship.

Mom played the piano and the accordion and had a beautiful voice. Chris's singing voice was a smooth tenor. When Chris first started learning to sing, Mom taught him to sing harmony, and they would sing for hours. Their music was the sound of home. I loved listening to them sing and talk and laugh.

Music was part of their deep bond. I never got the music gene, despite trying off and on for years to play the guitar, but I never felt jealous watching them play together. Mom had a deep and unique bond with all of us kids. We always felt deeply loved and secure when we were with her. Coming home always felt like a big, warm hug that touched your soul. Mom taught us how to love fully and unconditionally, that was her greatest gift.

Chris also had hemophilia, which ran in our family. It meant he was easily injured, and his body had a hard time stopping bleeding, internally or externally. He had to be extremely careful to avoid injury, but it was incredibly difficult, especially as a young boy. Everyday activities would put him in the hospital. Stepping off a sidewalk wrong, or bumping into a wall could start a bleed in his joints and that meant another hospital stay. Hemophilia can be excruciatingly painful, so they gave him strong painkillers, even as a toddler. He was diagnosed at two years old. It was difficult to manage not only the injuries, but the pain medication. Every time he was in the hospital, he was on strong narcotics, and then he had to get off pain pills when he came home. It wasn't easy for him or for our family.

One summer when he was around ten, he injured his knee again. This wasn't unusual; he often twisted his knee and ended up in the hospital. It was horribly swollen, at least doubled in size, and he couldn't bear to put any pressure on it. It was agonizing for him. His pediatrician told my mom to put him on the top bunk to force him to crawl down to use his knee. If he didn't, he told my mom he would be crippled.

I doubt that would be the approach today, but this was the '70s. Chris cried for hours. So did my mom. It was killing her to do that, but she did it. It was a horrible day. I felt helpless. I didn't really understand why Mom was being so mean, so cruel. Why wasn't she comforting Chris? She always made us feel better! Why not now? Why was she hurting him? I was only eight years old, and trying to make sense of this but just couldn't. After a while, I was so upset I had to go outside. I was in tears but wouldn't let Mom see that. She didn't need me crying, too. Before long, he climbed down, came outside, and we started playing. I was so happy! The three of us were incredibly close and when one hurt, we all did. That remained the case for our entire lives. I'm sure it was how I became so empathic. He ultimately regained full use of his knee. Looking back, I feel horrible for my poor mom who had to go against all her instincts as a mother to follow doctor's orders. She made some very tough decisions and, I'm sure, felt alone in having to do so.

Between Dad's drinking and Chris's health challenges, Mom didn't have much bandwidth left for me, let alone herself. I guess I always knew that and didn't want to add to it. I tried hard not to cause her any additional stress. I wasn't always successful, but I was a good kid. I didn't sneak out at night or skip school. Frankly, school was my happy place. I loved school. I felt safe and secure there. It was structured, and there were clear expectations. I thrived in that environment. At home, not so much. We never knew when Chris was going to get hurt or when Dad would start drinking. Or stop, for that matter. It wasn't always easier when he did stop, especially if he did it without getting treatment. Sometimes he could drink and stop at a few, but most times, it would turn into a week-long bender. He also worked shift work, so we had to be quiet while he was sleeping, which meant spending most of our time outdoors. It was like constantly walking on eggshells. Clearly, life at our house revolved around Dad, unless one of us kids was hurt, then, priorities shifted.

Chris wasn't the only one that gave our family scares. When Eric was eight years old, he was hit by a truck while riding his bike. I was cooking Cheeseburger Hamburger Helper for dinner. I remember because it was one of my favorites. I had been looking forward to it. He was badly hurt, and we weren't sure if he would make it. It was serious enough that they brought in a priest for last rites. He had broken his pelvis, ruptured his spleen, and there were a host of other issues that put him in critical condition. They kept a lot of the details from me, but I do remember being in the hospital and walking down the corridor to his room. I remember feeling fear and sadness from everyone around me. While Eric and I had our differences, (he could be quite annoying as only little brothers can), I loved him with all my heart. He was sweet and funny, and he was one of the Norling Mafia! We couldn't lose him. We wouldn't have survived the sadness and the heartbreak.

Mom rarely left his bed. Aunts and uncles were always there with us, helping us walk through that horrific event. They were there for Dad, too, but he had a hard time receiving love. Remarkably, Eric pulled through, and we could breathe again. We were used to hospitals because of Chris, but this was different. We had no frame of reference for what was happening to Eric. I never cooked nor ate Cheeseburger Hamburger Helper again. Ever.

Not surprisingly, I often felt invisible growing up. Part of that might have been because I was a middle child (there's been a lot written on that), but mostly it was because of the pressure I felt to not cause any additional stress on others. Usually Dad, Chris, or Eric demanded Mom's attention. I didn't have anything going on that could compete with them, so I spent a lot of time in my room. It was a bit of a vicious cycle. The more invisible I felt, the more I'd isolate myself in my room, and the more invisible I'd feel. I was sullen and prone to pouts. I know, it's not unusual for teenagers to act that way, but I always felt guilty because there were, literally, life-and-death situations happening all around me.

I was fully aware that Mom was at her wits end and I didn't blame her. Well, I probably did blame her in the way kids do, but I also understood there was a lot going on. I know that as a child, I shouldn't have had to worry about that, but I did, and it contributed to the dreads. I carried this behavior well into adulthood. It explains why it always made me uncomfortable to ask anyone to be inconvenienced. While I had no problem inconveniencing myself for others, asking others to do the same has always been extremely hard for me to do.

As a teenager, I had sullen down to a science. It drove my family crazy. On some level, I guess I knew that, and I would use it to manipulate them to get what I wanted. It forced them to pay attention to me. Sooner or later, they would ask me what was wrong. Finally, some attention!

Knowing what I know now, I feel bad about that, and I apologized to my mom years later. I knew no one had the energy to deal with whatever issue I was having (real or imagined), so I'd give everyone the silent treatment. I would take this strategy into adulthood. I was angry and hurt and feeling sorry for myself, so I made others suffer. Fair was fair, right? I would find out later that using silence to get people to pay attention to you, to see you, is a pretty rotten thing to do. I didn't learn that until late into adulthood, though. I'm sure I felt justified and maybe I was, as a child. In the end, it just added to my own guilt, so I'm not sure it was worth it.

I did my best to help Mom out by cooking, doing housework, and taking care of Eric when she was working. As soon as Chris was old enough, he was gone. He and Dad didn't get along most of the time, so the housework and chores fell to me from a young age. Personally, I didn't have a problem with doing chores. It gave me a lot of life skills that, at the time, weren't unusual to learn as a kid. Over time, though, more and more responsibility fell to me.

Sometimes, we would hit a good stretch when Dad was working and coming home on a regular basis to help out, but we couldn't depend on him to do that for long, especially in the early days before he quit drinking for good. Family members, especially Mom's sisters, would step in and help, so it wasn't always me carrying the burden, but enough of it fell to me that it was probably too much for a young girl. I did what I could, though. If nothing else, it sure taught me how to be self-sufficient.

I knew that whatever was going on with my family didn't define me. In all the craziness going on, my parents never made us kids feel like we caused any of it. We knew that wasn't on us.

I learned to grab on to the joy, no matter how small a sliver there was. I reveled in the calm when it was present, even though it usually meant Dad was off on a bender or in treatment. My favorite memories of my family are the mundane moments. Eating home-made cinnamon rolls at the kitchen table while the wood stove warmed the house during a snowstorm. Solving the world's problems together while washing the dishes. Listening to my brothers play music around the house. Those were special moments.

That's when Mom and I talked the most, often while doing dishes or canning. It's when she had the most bandwidth to breathe, and it's when we laughed the most. I realized early on that allowing myself to feel the good stuff helped balance out the bad stuff. I learned that from Mom. We just couldn't stay in the negative all the time. Any happiness and light we could find, that's where we went. I liked how I felt there. It took away the dreads. Maybe that's why I was always trying to find my way through; I knew the good stuff was on the other side.

Chapter Four

I knew how my world functioned within my family, even if it was unpredictable. The chaos became my comfort zone, and eating was my favorite coping mechanism. Like a lot of people, I stayed in my comfort zone out of fear, even when it wasn't a healthy place to remain. Early on, I lacked the skills to change how I experienced my life. Alcoholics Anonymous provided some tools, and I believe those helped me survive. However, I didn't have the bandwidth to thrive. I would later, but there was so much going on when I was growing up that getting through the day-to-day took a lot of effort. Just getting to school every day was a challenge. Navigating Dad's drinking and the minefield of our "normal" lives was exhausting. Even though I knew there was a different way, a more meaningful and fulfilling life out there, I stayed stuck, even into early adulthood. I was not stuck in the way of staying in the same physical space; after all, I left my home state of Michigan numerous times. However, how I approached life, how I made decisions, and more importantly, how I treated myself were as rigid as stone.

I had become quite comfortable thinking I was not worth extra effort or deserving of a better life. I made up all sorts of excuses as to why staying right where I was, mentally and emotionally, was good enough.

I told myself, *You don't deserve to have nice things. You want them but you can't have them because you don't look like everyone else. Look at you, you're lucky you even have the friends you have because of how you look.*

It all boiled down to, *It's okay to settle for this.* Was it really? Was it good enough because I was afraid or didn't know how to make the necessary changes to make my life what I wanted it to be? While no one ever told me I was stupid or deserved less than anyone else, I had somehow decided that was true.

Later, identifying why I was settling was key to figuring out the actions I needed to take to take back control of my life. Action can be a lot of things: taking a class, going to therapy, adding movement to your life, finding a coach, or reading a book about how to start a business. In a lot of ways, it doesn't matter where you start, the point is to take a step. Test the waters. Make a commitment to yourself to treat yourself better and to stop letting others determine the quality or trajectory of your life. You have so much more control over your life than you think you do. I promise that is true. Letting our circumstances define us is relinquishing our power to people who may not have our best interests at heart. I didn't know this for a very long time, but I finally figured it out. When I had suffered enough. When I had gone through enough. When I finally realized I deserved an amazing life, too. It would take me a long time to get there.

By the time I was in my mid-twenties, I was living at home and physically miserable. I should have been living on my own by then, but I just couldn't seem to make it happen. I was drinking way more than I should have been and making a lot of unhealthy decisions. I woke up one morning after a night of partying and felt awful. I was hungover, hanging out with people who I knew weren't good for me, and I was fat. I was embarrassed and disgusted. I wasn't sure what to do, but I had to do something.

The most obvious place to start seemed to be to lose weight. Isn't that where we always start? Isn't losing weight supposed to solve our problems? It never does, but it's where I started.

I joined a local weight loss program that had built-in accountability. It required maintaining a food diary, weighing and measuring portions, and checking in with coaches weekly. I do well when all those pieces are in place. The program wasn't anything revolutionary; I was eating lean protein, vegetables, fruit, and complex carbs. I started walking even though at the time, I couldn't walk a block without severe leg pain. After a while, the whole family was walking, sometimes up to ten miles a day on weekends. I had a lot of support, and everyone joined in. We supported each other's healthy habits, and all of us started to feel better. I didn't think to ask myself *why* I had been drinking so much and eating to excess. It didn't occur to me to even question that. I could fix the outside, though, and I did. I felt like a million bucks. I lost almost one hundred pounds and I felt great! I went from a size 20/22 to a size 10. Some people thought I was anorexic. Not even close. They just weren't used to seeing me at a relatively normal weight. In fact, I was still considered overweight, but I sure looked good!

However, college still eluded me. I had been going to college on and off for years. Periodically, I would move out of Michigan to spread my wings and give living on my own (or with a roommate) a try. Ultimately, I would end up moving back home. I just never seemed to get my life going. I felt as though I was never going to finish college at this rate. But I kept trying.

I was talking with a friend one evening, lamenting that at the rate I was going, I'd be thirty years old before I finished college.

"You're going to be thirty years old anyway," he said. "Do you want to be thirty years old with or without a degree?"

It finally clicked. It made perfect sense.

I believe God (or for others, the Universe) puts people in your path for many reasons, and one of them is to help you move forward when you're stuck. I've been blessed with so many of these people. The trick is recognizing when that is happening and being open to the gifts. Lord knows I've needed a lot of help along the way. We all do. I still do, more than ever. So, at age twenty-eight, I decided to go back to college and finish my degree for good. I was finally feeling better physically, so I had the energy and the focus to move on to other goals. I had accumulated about two years' worth of credits over the years, but still had no idea what I wanted to do, much less how to achieve it. I was going at it through trial and error the whole time. I had been successful at losing weight because the program gave me structure, discipline, and accountability. I realized, left to my own devices, I had no idea how to reach my goals. I needed the same structure, discipline, and accountability to finish school.

It had always made me feel inferior that I couldn't figure out how to graduate from college. My peers had all gone on to college and graduated in a reasonable amount of time, whereas I was taking one class a semester, passing some, failing others. I hadn't figured out how to study and take tests in college. It was a lot harder than high school. I found myself on academic probation a few times.

Sometimes, I couldn't take a class at all because I couldn't afford it. As a first-generation college student, I had no idea how to navigate the complex higher education system, and there weren't as many resources directed at my demographic at that time. I will give myself credit though, I never gave up, even though I had no idea how or if I would get to the finish line.

I didn't understand at the time that to reach any goal, you need to break it down into smaller, more achievable goals. My goal was to get a degree, that was it. I thought if I kept taking classes, sooner or later, I would graduate. That's not exactly how it works, though. There must be a plan, and you have to check a lot of boxes. It was confusing and overwhelming to me, and I didn't have anyone in my family who had even attempted to do this.

It was when I took a required class in public speaking that things started to click. I had found my place, my academic home. Accounting made no sense to me. Marketing? Nope. Forget about Chemistry, but Communication? I felt at peace and knew this was where I belonged. It made sense to me.

After that, there was no more academic probation. I finally started to gain traction. My grades drastically improved, and I felt like I was finally getting some academic success. It wasn't easy working and going to school, and I was frustrated at how long it was taking, but I was still committed to finishing.

If I had known the challenges I would face trying to graduate from college, I probably would have never started; it would have been paralyzing. However, I just kept moving forward, hoping what I was doing would, at some point, equal enough credits to graduate. I had been taking classes on and off for over ten years and was losing ground. My earlier credits were too old to count toward a degree, so I knew I had to make one final push if I was going to finish. One thing I knew for certain was continuing to lose ground wasn't going to help me graduate. The biggest hurdle at this stage was that I had no more money for college, and I was barely halfway to earning my bachelor's degree.

When I asked Dad if he would help me get a student loan, he said no. I didn't understand at the time why he refused, but it hurt my feelings that he had let me down once again. Mind you, Dad was supportive of my going to school but couldn't provide any financial support. Back then, Mom wasn't making much money so she couldn't help either. She felt bad about that. Later, she would pay for a summer class that allowed me to graduate on time. She was so proud she was able to help me. I'm sure Dad said no because he didn't understand how the process worked and knew he couldn't make that happen for me. His credit was probably shot. We'd already lost one house to foreclosure, and it wouldn't surprise me if there had been others.

I was pretty much on my own.

Despite that hurdle, I had my eyes set on New York University.

My cousin, Nancy LaMott, an amazingly talented singer, was already living in New York She and my mom were extremely close, so I knew her from her visits home. She always came by to see my mom, and they would eat Mom's homemade cinnamon rolls and drink tea. I flew to New York to visit NYU, spent some time with her, and got to know the city. Nan was in the recording studio when I arrived, so she sent a car for me. I thought I was quite special having a car service pick me up. I was dropped off at the studio where she was recording a demo for the upcoming Michelle Pfeiffer and Al Pacino movie, *Frankie and Johnny*. I walked in and sitting at the piano was Marvin Hamlisch. Nan introduced me as her cousin Gretchen and on the spot, Marvin wrote and sang a song about "Cousin Gretchen." It was one of the coolest things that had ever happened to me. Afterward, Nan and I joined some of her friends for dinner. And just like that, I fell in love with New York City. I submitted my application when I got home.

I had no idea how expensive it was to go to NYU, how much it would cost to live in New York City, or what I would do for a job once I got there (if I was even accepted). Why I thought I could get into one of the most prestigious private universities in the country was beyond me, though I always dreamed big. I knew I had turned my grades around and was a much stronger student now, but my college career in its entirety was less than stellar. I directly addressed my challenges in my personal statement; I didn't avoid it. Stories of overcoming adversity are powerful, especially if you're honest, own your part in it, and avoid excuses.

To my surprise, I was accepted! Perhaps they were impressed with my perseverance. Maybe they liked my story. Who doesn't want a student with that kind of fortitude? I'll never know what they saw in me, but I was going to NYU, and I was going to graduate! I just knew it! It helped that I received a generous scholarship. I was ecstatic! Nervous, but ecstatic.

I arrived at the Port Authority Bus Terminal in New York City in August 1991. It had taken two days on a Greyhound bus from Michigan. Nancy was singing in Atlantic City and left the keys with a neighbor. I schlepped my suitcases up a few flights of stairs to her apartment. It was a tiny studio on West 48th Street. If it was 300 square feet, I'd be surprised. I was only going to stay with Nan until I found somewhere to live.

You could call me all sorts of things—reckless, a dreamer, over-optimistic—but no one can call me a coward.

Fearless, I had no problem moving to New York without a solid plan. I had my acceptance letter and my suitcase. I figured the hard part was getting in, I'd just have to figure out the rest. Watch out world!

I found a job working at a large bank on Wall Street in the evenings and I secured some student loans. Between the two, I was doing ok. I ended up living with Nan, sleeping on a futon mattress on the floor.

I was in heaven.

All of a sudden, I had never felt so focused, so engaged, and so alive in my life.

Nancy was busy making records, and her career was really taking off. She had regular bookings at venues all over the city and beyond. She was doing performances on TV shows like *Live with Regis and Kathie Lee* and *Good Morning America*. I would go with her to some of her gigs and hang out with her glamorous, award-winning friends. I was having a blast. Between the two of us, we were as poor as church mice, but she was making it as a singer, and I was going to graduate from NYU. I never had a sister, so my relationship with Nan was special. Living together in New York, we became even closer. There were stark differences in our appearance. She was blonde, barely five feet tall, and I was a five-ten brunette. She had trouble reaching things on high shelves and when she needed my help she would call out, "Oh, tall person!" I don't know why that always made me laugh, but it did. Together, we were quite a formidable team.

NYU is in Greenwich Village, one of the most vibrant and diverse areas of the city. The energy was palpable. I was taking twenty credits at a time (I had to take a lot of classes to graduate in two years). Twelve credits were considered full-time, but you could take up to twenty credits for the same cost. I had no idea what I was getting myself into, but I thought it made the most sense money-wise to take the most credits I could.

I was thriving at NYU, earning top grades, working twenty hours a week at the bank, and loving life. I remember the first time I walked down to Broadway at midnight. The lights, the energy, the noise—it was intoxicating. I just stood there, taking it in. Listening. Watching. Smelling (trust me, there are a lot of smells in the city). New York is the only place I've ever lived where anything and everything was possible. People came from around the world to follow their dreams. If you were in New York, they could become reality. I was living a life that was truly beyond my imagination. I was starting to open my eyes to all sorts of possibilities and, for the first time, was building my confidence. Everything was in sync and momentum was building.

I love learning and school has always been my happy place. The first time I walked into Bobst Library at NYU, I was awestruck. It was huge! I just stood in the foyer and looked up. There were floors and floors of books. I love the smell of libraries, anyway, but this library? Holy smokes! I couldn't believe I got to come here anytime I wanted. To me, it represented knowledge and hard work. I spent hours upon hours in that library. I loved the smell of the old books. I loved the feel of the well-worn chairs made of sturdy wood, how they sounded when you moved them, and how they felt when you sat in them. It was like a warm hug, to me. I felt safe. I belonged there. Gretchen Norling, from Midland, Michigan was a student at one of the greatest universities in the country. Mind-blowing.

While at NYU, I approached every class with a sense of wonder and excitement, and I wasn't embarrassed about it. Being a non-traditional student had its drawbacks, but being excited to be sitting in that chair wasn't one of them. I understood the opportunity this was, and I wasn't going to phone it in. I never missed class, I was always prepared, and I studied hard. I asked questions and fully immersed myself in the culture of being a student. After making it to New York, I was never self-conscious again about being an older student. I embraced it. In fact, I celebrated it. I had worked so hard to make this happen; nothing was going to get in my way.

Once I was finally out on my own, I loved coming home. If I flew, I loved the moment when I walked through the gate and my mom or brothers would be waiting for me. Even though we had gone through so much as a family, there was no place like home, and I missed them when I was gone.

I talked to my mom every day on the phone. One Easter, I called Mom from New York because I was attempting to bake my first apple pie from scratch. My mom was known for her pies, but I had never really tried to make one myself. I must have called her ten times throughout the process. She was patient and so proud when it turned out. Since then, I've become a good pie maker and have taught a lot of people how to make them. I'll never be as good as my mom, but I can hold my own.

By my senior year, faculty were starting to talk to me about pursuing a PhD. I found that absurd. I hadn't even finished my undergraduate degree, and they were talking about me getting a PhD? I don't know what they saw in me, but they were watching me, nurturing me, and I loved the attention. They were investing in me. I had developed a reputation as a strong student and had something to contribute. They believed in me, and I was no longer invisible. They knew my name.

When I started out to get my degree the first time, I thought it was unattainable. I didn't think I would ever get there. I had so many obstacles and setbacks: finances, lack of discipline, lack of focus, little mentorship, and poor study skills. However, I never gave up. I kept working on each piece of the puzzle. It sometimes felt like one step forward and two steps back, but I never gave up. I was often frustrated, angry, disappointed in myself, and embarrassed because I couldn't manage to make it happen.

Now that I had found my discipline, found my academic home in New York, and was truly thriving, at least academically, not even finding the lump in my throat that turned out to be cancer would stop me, or even slow me down, once I saw the finish line.

Six months after I was diagnosed with thyroid cancer, I graduated from NYU. I couldn't believe it. I was graduating and magna cum laude at that! It took thirteen years, and I was thirty years old, but I was thirty years old with a college degree! Mom, Dad, and Eric came to New York for graduation and sat with Nancy to watch me cross the stage and receive my degree. The school-wide graduation was held outside in Washington Square Park, and it was a glorious day.

Wearing my purple graduation robe with my mortar board and tassel, I stood tall with my fellow graduates, one dot in a sea of purple. I enjoyed every second of the ceremony and all the other events that happened that week. I welcomed the congratulations and finally felt like I was even with my peers. I was so proud of myself.

We happened to be seated next to the celebrity tent. The actor, Alec Baldwin, had gone back to school to finish his degree so a lot of his friends and family were there. The coolest celebrity there, though? Neil Diamond. He was getting all the attention. I don't know who he was there to see, maybe it was Alec, but we all sat there staring at him. It was a magnificent moment, a true New York City experience. And then, when all the pomp and circumstance came to an end, I was officially a college graduate.

I felt complete, if only for a moment.

I thought getting a degree would provide stability and solve all my problems. In a lot of ways, I suppose it did, but what I didn't know then was that I had a lot of inside work to do to create the kind of life I wanted. Even more surprising, most of what I really wanted didn't have anything to do with a college degree or the number on the scale. It had a lot more to do with healing my traumas, reframing how I talked to myself, and believing that I deserved an amazing life as much as the next person. That would come much later. Unfortunately, I wasted a lot of time avoiding that work.

Chapter Five

After graduation, I flew back home to have the other half of my thyroid removed. I wanted to be around my family this time. Plus, I knew I would need to recuperate longer than I had for my first surgery. I was tired. The surgeries, finishing school, and the effects of thyroid cancer left me exhausted. My thyroid medication hadn't been adjusted correctly yet. I had gained all my weight back, my joints still hurt, and my body felt like it had been through a few rounds in the boxing ring. My endocrinologist was still in New York and because he would continue my follow-up care when I went back, I never had a conversation about RAI with anyone else. That would turn out to be a huge mistake.

While I was back, my family threw me a party to celebrate my graduation from NYU. It was filled with family, friends, food, and music. I was the first college graduate in our family, so this was a big deal. Dad and Mom were having problems again, but he was around for my party. My aunts, uncles, cousins, friends, and musicians all came to celebrate my graduation. It was mid-June, and the weather was perfect—blue skies and a slight breeze. There was so much food! Potlucks were a way of life in our family and this one didn't disappoint. There was also dancing and singing (many of Mom's side of the family were talented singers), and lots of laughter. It was wonderful catching up with everyone. When I came home for the holidays, I didn't always have time to see all my family and friends. When I look at the pictures from that day, I can still hear the laughter.

A few weeks later, Chris came down with some respiratory illness and wasn't feeling well. I came home and found him sitting in a recliner. He was obviously sick. He'd been to the emergency room and was given some medicine along with an inhaler to help him breathe. He told me he wanted to take a woman he cared for to Frankenmuth, a German-themed town, and asked me for $10. I gave it to him and kissed him on the forehead. I told him to get better, that I loved him, and that I'd see him later.

That was the last time I saw him.

They did go to Frankenmuth, and they danced to the sounds of an accordion in the parking lot. A few days later, he died of cardiac arrest. He was sleeping at my aunt's house and died in Grandma's old bed. He was thirty-two. My aunt, who was extremely close to Chris, had to make that phone call to tell Mom that he was gone.

Two years earlier, he had miraculously survived a car accident, which is a hemophiliac's worst nightmare. We had prepared ourselves to lose him then because he had to have emergency surgery, but he survived. We all thanked God for the miracle. While he was in the hospital, he talked to me about experiencing heaven and seeing God. Chris was a true believer, and I believed him. He asked me to find one of our local priests who he liked. My brother wasn't Catholic, but he had bonded with this priest. I don't know what they talked about that day, but he was a different man after talking with him. I suppose most people would be. It's hard to describe the change in Chris following that hospital stay, but he was more certain than ever that God existed, and that heaven was real.

Dad had not been home for a few weeks and Mom had a hard time finding him to tell him. In the meantime, we went over to see Chris before they took him away. He looked so peaceful lying in that bed. It was fitting that he died in Grandma's old bed. They were extremely close, and I'm sure she was there to welcome him. The night after Chris died, I crawled into bed with Mom. Just as I was falling asleep, I saw a bright light. He was finally home. Heaven gained a tenor.

We requested an autopsy. We didn't understand what had happened. We learned a couple of things. One, the cause of death was cardiac arrest due to the inhalant he'd been prescribed. And two, he was full of infection from a stitch that hadn't dissolved following his accident two years earlier. To be honest, it didn't matter why he died. He was way too young, and we knew we would feel that loss for the rest of our lives. We did. I still do.

The funeral was huge. All the musicians he'd played with or taught to play music over the years were there. I'd never seen so many young men wearing sunglasses. Everyone was having a hard time with this loss. Chris was well-loved. We found out later that while he never had any money to speak of, during the holidays he bought turkeys for families he knew were worse off than he was and left them on their doorsteps. None of us were surprised, because of course he did. The Christmas before he died, he didn't have much money, so he bought us all Bibles with our names engraved on them. He wrote a message to each of us and then proceeded to underline passages that meant something to him that he wanted us each to know. He wanted to make sure we understood the love Jesus had for us. I still have that Bible. Over twenty years later, Eric read those highlighted verses as part of my wedding ceremony.

We buried him at our family cemetery. That same year, my aunt would bury three of her five boys, all in their thirties, from complications of hemophilia and other diseases. That was the same year I was diagnosed with cancer and when Mom and Dad would finally divorce. It was a rough year.

That fall, I returned to New York. I knew at some point I was going to return to NYU to get a master's degree, and I knew it was time to start living again. I had finally figured out how to do this school thing. I wasn't done, not by a long shot. I was fully recovered from my surgeries and was feeling good. My life was moving forward again. Unfortunately, I had gained back all the weight I had worked so hard to lose a few years earlier. Thyroid issues, let alone cancer, will do that. When I was doing stand-up comedy, I always joked that I got the only cancer that makes you fat. It always got a good laugh. In real life, it wasn't all that funny.

I found work as an administrative assistant. The pay was good, but my heart wasn't in it. I quit and went back to NYU to pursue my master's degree. I loved graduate school. I was surrounded by people closer to my age, if not older. Collectively, we had more life experience that made our discussions more interesting. I didn't even care that our classes met until ten o'clock at night, which meant getting home close to eleven by subway. I'd use the time to reflect and be present, immersed in the moment. I was grateful to be back in New York City, living a life that was so vibrant and so full of color. I loved it.

That summer, I was able to secure a semester in England, studying at the University of London with amazing scholars. That was such a thrill for me and complemented my studies at NYU. I soaked up everything. I was becoming more confident in my ability to succeed. I was growing, maturing, and developing some much-needed confidence.

What I was still struggling with, of course, was my weight. An international flight in coach is uncomfortable when you're so overweight. Getting around London is hard when you have trouble walking long distances. Plus, there was still the issue of not liking the way I looked. It's one thing to be uncomfortable in your own body in a familiar place, but London was an entirely different culture with different people, and I was extremely self-conscious.

During my studies at NYU, there was one special professor, Dr. John Zimmerman, who made me work harder than anyone else. He pushed me way beyond what I thought I could do. He was the kind of teacher I wanted to become. He would come to class with half a dozen books, and he would read passages from each of them, all contradicting each other. Then we had to make sense of it all. I always left class with more questions than answers but also buzzing with energy. His approach made me think in more complex ways, something that wasn't easy for me. It was a whirlwind eighteen months, but I finished my master's quickly and was graduating again. This time, at Carnegie Hall.

When I walked across that stage, I stepped out of line to give Professor Zimmerman a big hug and to thank him for inspiring me to dream bigger. Mom and Dad were in the audience with a friend of mine. Mom told me later that night at dinner, that once she saw the doctoral candidates get hooded, she leaned over to my friend and said, "She's not done yet. She'll get her PhD." I didn't know that was going to happen, but she was right. Mom always was.

My evolution continued. I was becoming more intentional, and I liked how that felt. Professionally, I was starting to figure things out. I was working as a temp to make money, but I started to take control of my life and wasn't letting it just happen to me anymore. I was making a decent living in the city, but something was missing. I still wasn't quite sure what I wanted to do for a career, but I was getting closer. I could feel it.

Shortly after I started my master's, Nancy was diagnosed with uterine cancer. She was finishing what would be her final album. She delayed more aggressive treatment until she completed the album. She was working with the brilliant Peter Matz, who had worked with the best singers in the world, including Barbra Streisand. She finished the album in record time.

We spent as much time together as we could, and I was so grateful for the time we had. One evening when I was visiting her in the hospital, the phone rang. It was the White House. She had performed there twice for the then-sitting President Clinton and First Lady Hillary Clinton. Somehow, they found out she was sick and called her. I don't know what they said, but she perked up.

She said, "Hi, Mr. President," as I walked out of the room. What a moment for her.

Her cancer gave us another experience that we shared. We talked about what she was going through. I asked why she made the decisions she made around her cancer. She never asked me what she should do, that was between her and her doctor, but she admitted that she admired how I had handled my cancer journey. I made it clear that I was frustrated with her choice to go with less traditional medicine. I didn't think she had the luxury of experimenting to see if other approaches would work. Her body had been weakened over the years from Crohn's disease. She'd already had surgery that took a significant amount of her intestines and required her to have a colostomy bag. Her body was already severely compromised, yet she chose to start treatment by going to an alternative medicine healer. Her body, her choice. I just never understood the decision. By the time she decided to go a more traditional route, it was too late.

I remember being in the hospital when she had her colostomy surgery, and she was in so much pain. She was so small in that bed, and it was hard to watch her suffer. She was begging for stronger pain medication. They kept saying no. I argued with nurses and doctors constantly. In a moment of desperation, I yelled at them.

I was surprised they didn't kick me out. Understandably, the doctors were concerned about giving her more pain medication because of her petite size. They had every right to be worried about giving her too much. However, they didn't seem to understand that she'd been on incredibly high doses of narcotics for decades because of her Crohn's disease and had developed a very high tolerance. Somehow, I convinced them to raise the amount of pain medication, and I sat there for an entire day watching the clock so I could hit the self-administered pain pump the second it was time for more. Advocating for myself and my family came naturally, and I continued to advocate whenever Nan asked me to. She knew she could count on me.

Once we realized that she didn't have much time left, I called her family. I made sure they understood they needed to get here right away. I also called Mom. Given how close they were, I thought for sure she would want to be here. She didn't come. Perhaps she couldn't say goodbye to someone else she loved so dearly. I don't know, but Nan's dad, stepmom, and brother came and were able to spend her last moments with her. Shortly before she died, I had a few minutes with her alone. I told her how much I loved her, and she said the same. Her body was shutting down. She was cognizant but sleeping more.

"I'll fight with you as long as you want to fight," I told her, "But if you're tired, if it's time to go, it's ok."

I kissed her on the forehead and left. My heart hurt.

When I left the room, her friends Kathie Lee and Frank Gifford were in the hallway. That's when I first met them. They were very sweet. Nan had been recuperating at their house in Connecticut following her chemotherapy treatments. I was grateful that they took such great care of her.

She'd been dating a great guy, and they wanted to be married. We all knew she didn't have much time left, so they were married at the hospital and a few hours later, Nan died.

She was forty-three.

Another family member too young to die. She had become more and more successful just before she died. She had been on numerous TV shows and developed quite a following. In fact, there was a story about her in the tabloid *The Star* when she died. It highlighted Kathie Lee Gifford's relationship with Nan and how she had lost a good friend. Nan would have loved that, her tabloid debut.

I miss her so much.

Her music lives on, though, and I listen to it often. I especially like it when she talks or laughs before she starts singing. I hate that she's gone, but it's comforting to be able to listen to her whenever I want to.

Around this same time, I was also in the midst of getting divorced from my short-lived first marriage. I realized it was time to move on. As much as I loved it, it was time to leave New York. It had finally clicked that getting my PhD was what I wanted to do, and it was getting too expensive to stay in New York. Even though I would be forty years old when I graduated, I knew that's what I had to do.

I had no idea if I *could* do it, but I thought if everyone else thought I could do it, then I could. I remembered what my friend had told me when I was struggling to finish my undergraduate degree, and just applied the logic forward a decade. I was going to be forty years old anyway. Might as well be forty and have a PhD.

By then, I also knew what I needed to study. I searched for programs that would combine my interests in communication and health.

Health issues were pervasive in my family, and I wanted to study something that I could apply in my own life. With every major health crisis—Chris's hemophilia, my cancer, Nan's cancer, even Dad's alcoholism—came struggles in communicating with doctors and medical professionals.

Frankly, I wanted some answers, and I wanted to understand why they were sometimes so hard to get. Health Communication was the perfect fit. I applied to two programs: one in Michigan and one in Kentucky. I was wait-listed at Michigan State University and was accepted to the University of Kentucky in Lexington, Kentucky. I was ready to go. I had $113 in my pocket the day I left

New York. I had secured graduate student housing, so at least I had somewhere to live.

It was another huge step towards defining my life and shaping it the way I wanted it to be. We can use our experiences as catalysts to make our lives better, or we can let them have power over us for the rest of our lives and settle. I was finally done settling. I know for a fact that I have the power to do the work necessary to minimize the effects of my childhood. I can use those experiences to make me stronger, more empathic, and more compassionate. I am who I am because of my family, but the story doesn't end there. It's only where I started. I realized I had to own my story, because let's be honest, denial doesn't help anyone. I also had to figure out what I wanted in life and do the work to make it happen.

Simple, right? Sure.

Easy? Not so much.

Chapter Six

I arrived in Lexington, Kentucky in August of 1998. My divorce was finalized, and I looked forward to starting school again. I couldn't believe I would be a doctoral student at one of the top programs in the country. I was nervous, for sure, but I had gained confidence over the past few years and felt this was where I was supposed to be. The slower pace of Lexington would be a better environment for going to school. Plus, it was only an eight-hour drive to Michigan, much closer to my family than I'd been in New York. It meant I could see my family more. They loved coming to Lexington, especially Eric.

My health was relatively stable. My blood work showed that my cancer was still gone, but my weight was still out of control. I was one hundred pounds overweight and as anyone will tell you, eventually you just hurt. Not only could I not be as physically active as my friends and colleagues; it took all I had to get through the day. I never did get my second wind back after I had my cancer surgery. Every few years, I would try to lose weight by restricting calories or joining a gym, but it never stuck. My approach was always too extreme. I'd get to a point when I was disgusted, usually because someone rejected me or made fun of me, and I'd decide to do something. That was always short-lived, but I never gave up entirely.

Over time, a pattern emerged. I would decide to do something about my weight. I would be successful for a while, and then I would quit. I would become completely hopeless and resign myself to a life of being overweight. That would last for a few months until I could give it another try. I would do something extreme again. I would fail. I would feel hopeless and beat myself up because I was weak and had no willpower. Then, I would do it all over again. I wish I had known earlier that losing weight had nothing to do with willpower so I would stop beating myself up. I didn't, and every time I failed, I berated myself more.

Lexington was another fresh start. A new city. New possibilities. A new me.

I loved Lexington from the start. It's a beautiful city with vibrant food and culture. I didn't have a car, having just moved from New York City, so I had to rely on my new friends to pick me up if we were doing anything. I did do some proactive planning, something I was proud of myself for. I was worried about being lonely in a new town. To avoid sitting around and feeling sorry for myself on Saturday night, which I was prone to do, I arranged to volunteer in the emergency department at the hospital. I chose the 8-11 p.m. shift. It was one of the smartest things I'd ever done. Not only did it keep me busy every Saturday night, but it made me feel good to be helping patients or families who needed a friendly face during a scary or long night in the emergency room. I only did that one semester because I was plenty busy the next term, but I still am grateful that I had the forethought to do that.

Periodically, Eric would come and stay with me for a while. I liked having him around. He made me laugh. Navigating a doctoral program is stressful, and he distracted me by forcing me to get out and experience more of what Lexington and the surrounding areas had to offer. Actually live a little. It's easy to make your world very small when you're in a doctoral program. It's always demanding your attention, and there's always an overabundance of work to do, so it was good for me to take breaks. We would go to concerts and bluegrass festivals. Sometimes we'd just go for long drives. I loved the time we spent together.

To stay on top of my health, I was getting blood work done, as directed. So far, so good. There was no evidence of the cancer returning. For some ridiculous reason, I decided to fly to New York every six months for follow-ups. I'm not sure how I thought I'd be able to afford that as a doctoral student, but that was the plan. So that's what I did for a while.

In the meantime, my weight was the highest it had ever been. Between Nan's death, my divorce, moving to a new city, going to school, and trying to navigate life in general, I kept eating. That had always been my go-to coping strategy and nothing had changed. I had plenty to be stressed about, and my health showed it. I felt awful. It's not easy moving around in a body that's so big. My feet always hurt from plantar fasciitis, and I just looked and felt generally bad. I didn't have a thyroid anymore and while synthetic thyroid hormones do a good job of keeping you alive, I never felt 100%. I was always tired, and I never had anything extra in the tank. I didn't let it stop me from doing what I had to do, but it sure made life harder than it needed to be.

Being a doctoral student was surreal. I had no idea what it would entail or how to approach it. None of us did. I lucked out, though. I was part of the most amazing cohort of doctoral students. We bonded immediately. I remember saying on day one that we would need to lean on each other to get through this. No one was going to survive it alone. It's long and arduous. The coursework is relatively manageable compared to the qualifying exams and the dissertation, but it's still a marathon and there are plenty of ways to get derailed. While you have a committee that guides you, you still have to do the work. It's a highly self-directed process. No one comes to your house to make sure you're writing or analyzing your data. It's on you. At least, I was smart enough to put together the most rigorous committee I could from the beginning. I figured that way, if I finished, I'd know what I was doing.

I was studying health communication and there was no better place to do that than at the University of Kentucky. It had (and still has) one of the most respected health communication programs in the country. To this day, I'm not quite sure how I got in.

I knew I was interested in provider-patient communication because I'd had so many terrible interactions over the years. Frankly, I wanted to figure out why it was so bad. The medical visit was highly dependent upon providers and patients being able to communicate, and based on my life experience, that wasn't happening very effectively. I not only wanted to figure out why it wasn't working but, more importantly, how to fix it.

There are always multiple paths through a doctoral program (life, too, for that matter). You can take the path of least resistance, do the bare minimum, and still earn a PhD. Or you can take a more rigorous path and push yourself harder than you think you can stand. I took the latter path. As fate would have it, I was assigned to one of the most talented and respected scholars in health communication as an advisor/mentor, Dr. Nancy Harrington. I was a year older than Nancy, which made me a little more comfortable, I suppose. I guess it should have made her a little less intimidating, but that's not how it felt at the time. She was tough, and she oversaw the entire department as its chair. She had incredibly high standards and expected everyone to meet them. I did my best from day one, but that's not to say I was always successful. I asked her to be my dissertation chair, and she agreed. There aren't a lot of hard and fast rules about navigating this process, and I made the mistake of writing my proposal without her guidance. I had worked with another committee member on it and felt certain she would be impressed with my initiative and brilliant writing. She wasn't. I had to start over. I was mortified, but I learned my lesson.

No surprises.

I remember meeting with her to go over the first few chapters of my dissertation. I had turned it in for her comments, and when she handed it back to me there wasn't a single sentence that didn't have edits on it. It was a sea of red marks. I may have been able to keep a few words here and there. *Holy smokes,* I thought to myself, *this is going to be way harder than I anticipated.* I never had to write a master's thesis at NYU, so this was all new to me. From the beginning of my doctoral studies, I always felt a little behind, and I had to work extra hard to maintain my grades. While I had written a lot of papers at NYU, I wasn't as skilled in scholarly writing as I should have been. Getting a C in graduate school pretty much means you failed, so I did everything I could to get an A. I did get a B once. It was in statistics. Considering I had absolutely no prior experience with the subject, I was good with it.

I continued to work and rework my chapters and one day while meeting with her, I noticed an entire page with no edit marks on it. None. At the bottom of the page was a smiley face. I'd never been so proud. I was transforming into a serious doctoral student and was emerging as a leader. I was also finally realizing that being seen and heard was critically important to me. I felt I had something to contribute to the world and for the first time, my life experience, including the good times and especially the bad times, had value. It was why my perspective was important. I was coming at the subject from a place of real-life experience. I was finding my voice in the world of academia, and it was getting louder. I was very much coming into the light. My soul was soaring.

Earning your PhD can be brutal. You're exhausted, you constantly doubt yourself, and at some point, you realize you're never going to get it all done. Frankly, it all feels impossible. Some days you're teaching classes or working as a research assistant; other days you're taking classes; and in between it all, you're doing homework, reading journal articles, writing papers, grading assignments, and trying to figure out what your dissertation needs to focus on. I was working all weekend, sleeping little, and eating whatever I could easily find. Convenience made it very carb-heavy. No one I knew ever turned to a salad when they were stressed, and neither did I. Graduate school was filled with lots of food and drinking.

Every Tuesday night was trivia night for my cohort and that meant bar food and alcohol. Not surprisingly, I was gaining even more weight. It's not the healthiest time of anyone's life, I'm sure. Probably one of the healthiest things I did was grocery shopping. I didn't have a car for the first year, so I had to walk a couple of miles to the grocery store. I had brought my shopping cart from New York, so most weekends found me pushing it to Kroger and walking back with a cart full of groceries. I'm sure I looked ridiculous, but it was the only way to get groceries. As a relatively poor graduate student, cabs were a luxury I couldn't afford. Sometimes, one of my friends would take me grocery shopping. After a year or so, I realized I had to buy a car. I had finally secured a research assistant job and could finally afford one.

I threatened to quit my PhD program a few times. The first time was after I had finished writing my qualifying exams. I had completed my coursework, and it was time to prove to my committee that I was ready to do my dissertation. I had just spent five days writing non-stop in the library and had written over sixty pages for the five questions I was given by my committee. I went to Nancy's office to hand in my answers.

"I'm quitting," I told her, handing her the pages.

She looked up at me. "No, you aren't. Go home and take a nap. I'll see you on Monday."

"No," I insisted, "Really, I quit."

She reiterated that I was not quitting and told me to go get some rest. I just stood there looking at her for a minute. I was so tired. I went home and took a nap.

I didn't quit.

I was an anxious wreck over having to orally defend what I had just written, and Eric, who was visiting me at the time, asked why I was doing this to myself. I was crying from the stress. His question stumped me. I couldn't tell him why I was putting myself through this, I just knew I needed to prove to myself that I could do it. I wanted this. This is what I wanted to do. I wanted to be a professor. I wanted to be an academic. I also think part of it was because, for the first time, I would feel like I not only caught up with my peers but surpassed them. I would be ahead for the first time, whatever that even meant. There was also great honor and prestige attached to earning a PhD. I wanted to experience that.

Throughout my educational process, I was finding my voice. I was healing from feeling invisible growing up. I was finding that I was worthy of whatever I wanted to be or do. Even though I was exhausted, I was smiling more and was happier than I'd ever been. I was learning that I was smart. I was respected. I was finally clearing my path to my future.

Chapter Seven

In April of 2000, I woke up one morning and the first thing that popped into my head was, *Get to the doctor.* I had no symptoms beyond being tired, which I attributed to being a PhD student. We were all exhausted. Overall, I was feeling fine. My blood work was normal. Still, the voice was strong. To this day, I believe it was my older brother, Chris. After his death, I could still feel his spiritual presence. I have a lot of angels around me, but Chris was my big brother, and he always had my back when he was alive. Apparently, that hadn't changed in death. Years later I would tell this story to other physicians and every one of them said they couldn't explain it, either. Whatever the explanation, I called the University of Kentucky Markey Cancer Center the next day. I needed to find a specialist who treated thyroid cancer. There was one. One. I thought, *Oh, Lord. Where am I? There's only one doctor to choose from? Heaven help me.* It turned out that he was one of the leading thyroid cancer doctors in the country. Once again, I was in the right place at the right time and the right people appeared in my life.

When I met with him, we talked about my history of thyroid cancer. I explained that I had had two surgeries to remove both lobes of my thyroid; however, I had never been treated with I-131 radioactive iodine (RAI). He was furious, not at me, but at my medical team. It made absolutely no sense to him that I had not received the standard treatment for thyroid cancer the first time. There should have been no question about it. It was absolutely what should have happened. It didn't.

He ordered the same bloodwork that I had been doing for the past seven years, which had always shown everything was normal. He ordered nuclear scans to see what, if anything, was going on. I remember going into his office with my mom. She was in town to be with me when I got my results.

He looked at me and said, "I'm sorry to tell you, the cancer is back. Plus, it's spread to your lungs."

I was not prepared to hear that news. I was in shock. Mom was in shock. I had no symptoms. I asked how that could be given my bloodwork has always been normal. He explained that a small percentage of the population doesn't respond to those tests. He said that by the time anything showed up in my bloodwork, the prognosis would not be very good at all. The cancer was spreading. The hope was, because the metastases were only a light dusting that the cancer would respond to aggressive treatment. It was painfully clear that I should have received the standard treatment during my first bout of thyroid cancer. I didn't. Now I was going to pay dearly for it.

The thing about a cancer diagnosis is that once you hear you have cancer, it's difficult to process what is said next. The same is true the second time. The doctor discussed what would happen, but neither my mom nor I comprehended it. I would find out weeks later via email, when I finally had the wherewithal to even ask what stage cancer I had, that it was Stage 4. I didn't share that with anyone, including my family. People knew I had cancer, but not the specifics. I didn't want them to worry. It was my default behavior since childhood to not give my family anything more to worry about, especially my mom. I justified it by the fact that at no point did I think I would die from it. Why scare them? I don't know why I didn't think I would die when I absolutely could have. I just didn't.

When you are diagnosed with cancer, there are multiple dynamics occurring simultaneously. Obviously, when you have cancer (or any serious illness, for that matter), the focus is on treatment and getting through it successfully. But the dynamic people don't often talk about is how the person who is sick has to balance navigating their illness and treatment with interacting with their loved ones. It's excruciatingly difficult and emotionally draining to look at the faces of your parents, siblings, children, or friends and loved ones and see their worry. I recently heard a cancer survivor call them "sad eyes." Sad eyes, indeed.

I was incredibly close to my family, especially my mom. I greatly admired her. She was the strongest, wisest woman I knew. She had navigated and survived extremely difficult obstacles, and yet she still lit up the room when she walked through the door. To say my mom was special doesn't even begin to describe how amazing she was. I was also extremely close with Eric. Since Chris died, it was just the two of us kids, and we grew closer and closer as time went on. He was my best friend and my hero.

The doctor explained the treatment plan again at my next visit. I was more prepared to hear what he had to say then. He mentioned something about dosimetry. I had no clue what that was. He explained that he had to determine how much radioactive iodine my body could handle before it basically shut down my immune system. He was known for being aggressive in thyroid cancer treatment. Thankfully, I had him in my corner.

To receive the radioactive iodine, I had to be taken off my synthetic thyroid medication and put on a shorter-acting medicine so that it would all be out of my system by the time I went into the hospital for treatment. This, along with a low-iodine diet, makes the cancer cells hungry for iodine and they absorb the treatment more effectively. We also needed the radioactive iodine to bypass my neck and travel to my lungs. There were no guarantees that it would. It depended on how successful my previous surgeries were. Did they get the entire thyroid and surrounding tissues, or did they leave some? We would soon find out.

Coming off the medication was a painful process. It's not that I went through withdrawal in the typical sense, like with pain medicine, but it was debilitating. The thyroid is an important gland; it regulates your metabolism, heart rate, blood pressure, and body temperature. Too much thyroid hormone causes hyperthyroidism, which causes irregular or rapid heartbeats and weight loss, along with lots of other serious health problems. Too little, which was my issue, causes important functions to become stressed in a different way. Hypothyroidism causes fatigue, heavy menstrual cycles, difficulty thinking, muscle weakness, muscle and joint pain, and a host of other issues.

The whole process took about six weeks to prepare for treatment. For the first month, I just felt a little tired because the medicine I was taking to replace my thyroid medication did a good job. However, the last two weeks before treatment, I had to stop taking the medication altogether. Now I had no thyroid hormone in my body at all. Boy, did I start feeling that. I was in the middle of my PhD program, still taking classes, and doing my best to work as a research assistant. At some point, though, I paused it all to focus on treatment.

After I stopped taking all my medication, I started experiencing severe joint and muscle pain along with peripheral neuropathy (my feet started to go numb which, strangely enough, is very painful). I also was experiencing brain fog. Everything started getting confusing; I couldn't concentrate at all. This is not a good thing when you're doing coursework for a PhD program! I was also having trouble getting in and out of bed. I couldn't stand long enough to cook, and I couldn't drive because of the effects of having no thyroid hormone in my body. My reflexes were extremely slow. I was in a lot of pain, and my system needed to stay clean for the scans, so no pain medication was prescribed. I have no doubt that this was exacerbated by my weight. Our weight impacts everything related to our health in some way. I'm not saying it's the only thing, but it played a role.

Eric came down to stay with me to cook and help me get around. As part of the preparation for treatment, I was put on a zero-salt diet to remove all traces of iodine from my system. Absolutely no salt, which meant everything had to be made with fresh meat, fresh vegetables, and fresh fruit which meant nothing canned, nothing pre-made, and no restaurants or fast food. You would be amazed at how much salt is in seemingly healthy food. We became experts at reading labels. Eric got creative with his menus. He perfected a breakfast sausage recipe that tasted exactly like what we grew up eating in Michigan. I was really missing eating toast, so Eric made multiple attempts at no-salt-added bread but that didn't turn out so well. I couldn't have done it without him. He stood steadfastly by my side as I became sicker and sicker waiting for my scans. A few days before going into the hospital, I could only get out of bed to go to the bathroom. Even that took considerable effort and assistance. Eric never flinched. I can only imagine what he was thinking as he helped me to the bathroom. But he did that and whatever else needed to be done. That's how we always were with each other. Whatever had to be done, no matter how uncomfortable, we did it. We never left each other to fight anything alone. We were always there for each other.

Eric always made me laugh. He was my little brother, and he was my rock. Still, I never told him I was Stage 4. My thought was that if the first round of treatment didn't go well, I would tell my family how serious it was, but, if it was successful, my decision to withhold that detail would be justified. Our family had experienced so much health-related stress in our lives that I didn't have the heart to add to it. Unless it was necessary to tell them, I wasn't going to.

I was admitted to the hospital and put in isolation. Normally, you aren't hospitalized for RAI, except in rare cases when you are receiving extremely high doses. I was going to get a very high dosage. The goal of RAI is to kill all the remaining thyroid cancer cells so they can't spread to other parts of your body. That's why I should have gotten RAI when I was first diagnosed and had my initial surgery. I would have received a small dosage following my surgery and wouldn't have had to be hospitalized at all. It would have been a breeze. It certainly wasn't a breeze now. What would have been no big deal a few years prior had now become a very big deal.

Being in isolation was, well, lonely. There was a piece of colored tape on the floor in my room and no one, except my doctor, was supposed to cross that line. I wasn't allowed visitors so I could only talk to my family and friends by phone. I was nervous, scared, and alone. My doctor explained what was going to happen, but I don't think anyone is able to truly comprehend what treatment for any serious illness entails. There were so many details and when your cognitive function is impacted, the complex details become even more difficult to understand. I just put one foot in front of the other and whatever the next step was, I did it. I didn't think that far into the future, not because I didn't think I had one, but because it was all so overwhelming. Thank God I had my family to help me navigate this journey, I couldn't have done it without them. Even with all our dysfunction, it's what Mom, Eric, and I did for each other. Dad was another story. He tried but he wasn't always successful. I knew he loved me but wasn't sure he could face it.

The radioactive iodine treatment was delivered by a man wearing what looked like a hazmat suit, and he was wearing huge gloves. He looked like an astronaut. He stood behind the line on the floor which meant I had to get out of bed and walk over to him. Using long tongs, he took the pill out of a small metal container and handed it to me. He told me I had to swallow it. I was thinking, *He can't even touch this thing, and I have to swallow it?* I swallowed it.

Shortly thereafter, I had my nuclear scans and was allowed to start back on my thyroid medication. I was never so happy to start taking medication in my life. It would take six to eight weeks to get back to normal, but I felt better almost immediately. I'm sure part of that was mental, but I didn't care. I could go back to school and eat a regular diet.

I remained in the hospital for a few days until my radioactivity levels were acceptable. Turns out, it's a public health hazard to have radioactive people walking around, so I had to stay in isolation until I was safe to be around. After I went home, I had to keep my distance from people for a few weeks, but being home was a lot better than being in isolation. I started feeling so much better. Eric was still staying with me and made sure I was on the mend before he went back home. Having him there meant the world to me.

There were no guarantees that the radioactive iodine would work. Did it travel all the way through my body to reach my lungs? I would have to wait six months before I could be scanned to see if it worked. In the meantime, I was ready to get back to my life as a PhD student.

My professors, fellow students, and my dissertation chair, Nancy, were wonderful during this process. Nancy had a lot on her plate, but she made sure I was ok and checked in regularly. I didn't talk a lot about it, but she knew what was going on, and she helped me navigate this difficult time. I don't know whether the faculty had much experience with students going through Stage 4 cancer treatment, but they were very understanding and supportive. I was and remain grateful they stood by me throughout my cancer journey.

About six months later, I was taken off my medication again and put back on the salt-free diet, in preparation for the nuclear scans to see if the treatment worked. Eric came back down to help me again. He knew the drill. We were a pretty good team, and we had the process down to a science. I still didn't tell anyone I was Stage 4.

I honestly don't know how I kept it from my family. Normally my mom could tell when something was on my mind from just looking at me. It probably stemmed from when I was a little girl. She once told me that my eyes turned a different color when I lied, so I would never look at her if I was lying. Obviously, a huge tell. It was a pretty smart tactic if you ask me. She was in Michigan, and I was in Kentucky. Primarily talking on the phone. I was able to hide it. I never said a word. I think part of it was because I was convinced that I was going to be alright.

In retrospect, it wasn't fair to them. Admittedly, it's not easy for families to watch their loved ones go through cancer treatments, but people don't always realize the burden it places on the sick person to watch their loved ones so scared. At some point, you become more concerned with how they are feeling than how you are healing. At least I did.

Parents who are sick have to decide when and if they should tell their young children, and if so, how much to share. Adult children have to decide how much to tell aging parents. Siblings? Close friends? It's hard to know. While family and friends may feel entitled to know, ultimately, only you can decide what to do in your situation. It may have been selfish to withhold the information but, at the time, it seemed like the right thing to do. We always tried to protect each other in our family, especially Mom, Eric, and me. Looking back, I should have told them from the beginning. They were incredibly hurt when I finally told them; they felt betrayed even though they understood my reasoning. Either way, they were going to be hurt, and I guess I felt I would rather have them mad at me than worried about me. To this day, I'm not convinced my strategy was justified. Truthfully, I really needed to talk about having Stage 4 cancer with them, to help me process it, and I denied myself that by not telling them. I carried most of that burden alone. It's one of the biggest regrets I have, and I promised I would never do it again. I lied.

When you do nuclear scans, you lie on a very narrow table. They tape your head and strap your body tightly to the table so you can't move a muscle. I had to have multiple scans that would take up to forty-five minutes each and for the entire time, I couldn't move. I couldn't even scratch my nose, and my back was killing me. I was still morbidly obese, which made it even more uncomfortable. The table was probably ten inches wide, and I was way wider than that. It was so uncomfortable, and even though the staff would do everything they could to make me as comfortable as possible, everything hurt.

My body hurt from not having thyroid hormones in my system. It also hurt from being strapped in for so long on a hard table. It just hurt. My body had to remain completely still, or I would risk having to repeat the scans. I would lie there for hours with small breaks when I could finally bend my knees. I've never had a baby, but I understood that deep breathing could help get you through almost anything. I focused on my breathing the entire time. It helped quell my anxiety and fear.

Lying on that table for that long gave me a lot of time to think. This was my second bout with cancer. The first time didn't seem like a very big deal, just as everyone kept telling me. I was lucky to get "the good cancer." I never understood how anyone could think getting any cancer wasn't a big deal. They may have been trying to make me feel better but, later, I realized it minimized my experience and what I was going through. I guess I let people do that because I didn't know how to respond when they said that. My family never said that, but there were plenty of others who did. Obviously, they didn't understand how much having cancer of any kind affects your life. Frankly, I wouldn't understand the full extent until much later. However, it definitely got my attention this time.

The first time I became a cancer survivor, I didn't think that much about it. I was grateful I was okay, but I didn't think it had impacted my life that much in the short term, so I just carried on. It did change how I talked about myself. I was vocal about having had cancer and identified as a survivor, but I always felt guilty (and still do) because I didn't have to go through extensive treatments or suffer the significant side effects that often accompany the disease. I never had any outwardly visible signs that I had cancer. No significant weight loss (in fact, I experienced the opposite), no hair loss, and no chemotherapy or radiation. The second time I had cancer it changed me in profound ways. First, it impacted me physically, and even twenty-plus years later, it still does. I deal with the effects of my thyroid cancer treatment every day. Due to the damage to my salivary glands, I have trouble swallowing (I also have Sjogren's Disease which causes dry mouth, so it's probably a combination of the two). That means I must be extremely careful when I eat because I choke easily. That's why I always, and I mean always, carry water with me. Everywhere. The simplest food can make me choke. Having diminished salivary gland production means you can't break down your food like you should in order to swallow. I must be mindful at all times. It makes me feel old. The aging process weighs heavily on my mind, and I worry about it.

About ten years post-RAI treatment, I started having dental problems due to my perpetual dry mouth and found myself in the emergency room multiple times with tooth abscesses. I have had to have multiple teeth pulled since, resulting in dental implants. The problem continues today. The sad part was if I had known to tell my dentists about my thyroid cancer and treatment, I could have avoided all of this by using prescription toothpaste. No one ever asked, and I didn't think to tell them. I also don't have a second wind anymore. Once my energy is gone, it's gone. You can watch me shut down. My face gets pale, my eyes become dull, and I'm just done. I have to rest and recharge. My mom could always tell the second I was out of energy. Sometimes, she knew before I did.

Cancer changes how you look at and talk about yourself. I was now a two-time cancer survivor. It forces you to take stock of your life. I know it's cliché, but it's true. The world keeps spinning, but your perspective changes. You're a member of a club no one wants to join. I started thinking about what I should do having made it through cancer twice. To be honest, I didn't know what I was going to do differently, but I knew things were not going to be the same. It wouldn't be until my third bout with cancer that I would truly make the changes I needed to live a more intentional life. I guess I'm a slow learner.

I'm still surprised I finished my PhD on time. After treatment, I went back to normal life as a doctoral student, meeting all of the milestones and, ultimately, successfully defending my dissertation. Life was good. My energy level never completely returned, but I couldn't tell at the time if that was cancer or graduate school. Either way, I went on with my life. I wasn't entirely healthy, but I was cancer-free. I graduated with my PhD at forty years old. When I got hooded, Mom, Dad, and Eric were there.

Chapter Eight

About a year after I had completed my PhD, I had the opportunity to go to Prato, Italy to present my research at a conference. I was so excited to visit Italy. Some friends of mine from New York were visiting at the same time and they invited me to stick around and stay with his family in a small town outside of Florence. I didn't hesitate and extended my ticket.

It was a magnificent experience. I was in my early forties, and I realized that I tended to always be looking toward the future, seeing what was next, and never truly being content in the present. In Italy, I focused on slowing down and enjoying the moment. The food was exquisite. I had dinner one evening with my friends and their family. There were eight or ten of us sitting outside under the stars eating food that was all grown locally. The meat, the cheeses, the olive oil, the bread, and the wine, it was amazing! It was unlike anything I'd ever experienced before. I only spoke English, which limited my interaction, but everyone tried so hard to include me. I was hooked. I had decided that when I got back, I would buy a one-way ticket to Italy. As usual, I had no plan, but I was sure that's what I needed to do.

When I returned to the States, I bought that ticket and planned to move to Italy that summer once my job ended. Of course, I had no idea how to move to another country. I didn't have a clue about Visa requirements, or if I could even move to another country legally, or how to get a job. As usual, I just thought I'd wing it and figure it out as I went. In the meantime, another opportunity came up. I was working as a visiting assistant professor at the University of Pittsburgh when I was contacted about an assistant professor position at The University of West Florida. I was so torn. I desperately wanted to move to Italy, but this was a fantastic opportunity that I couldn't turn down. As was my pattern, I hadn't told my family I was planning to move to Italy, though I'm sure that wouldn't have surprised anyone.

I accepted the job at UWF. When I told Mom and Eric I was moving to Pensacola, Florida, they decided they'd join me if I was open to it. We would all share a house. Mom was retiring and Eric hadn't been working for a while due to his back issues. I thought it was a great idea. I loved the time we spent together. I had been gone for so many years; it was healing to be with one another. To be honest, I always had trouble leaving my family when it was time to go.

While I loved living in different cities, especially New York, I cried every time I had to leave my family. It didn't matter how old I was, I got emotional. I missed my mom and my brother. I missed Dad, too, but my relationship with Dad was more complicated. We talked on the phone, and I usually saw him when I was home, but it was for shorter periods of time. But I spent every waking moment I could with Mom and Eric. We rarely made plans, even if I came home for the holidays. We just relished the time we had together. After Chris died, we understood time was a precious commodity. It took Eric years to process losing Chris, and I suppose he never really recovered. We talked about Chris all the time. I still do.

It took Mom a long time to re-engage at the holidays once Chris was gone. It was so hard on her. I can't imagine burying your child.

It's not the natural order. That may be why we were so protective of our time together when I came home. We just wanted to be close without distractions. Sometimes, no one else even knew I was home because it got so chaotic trying to see everyone. Frankly, I really just wanted to be with Mom and Eric. I think Dad had the worst time over losing Chris, though. He had horrific guilt, and we'll never know how much that ate him up inside.

I wanted to see my relatives, but I was usually so tired that all I wanted to do was rest and take naps. Taking naps at Mom's was the only time I could truly relax and shut my mind off. I felt safe there. I knew everything was going to be okay when I was home. The hardest decision I'd have to make was what we were going to have for dinner. I think that's why having the opportunity to live together again was so important to me. I'm sure not everyone could do that, but we could, and it was, in retrospect, a sacred time. A gift.

Once we got settled in Pensacola, I decided, once again, that I needed to lose weight and get healthy. I was at my highest weight and in my mid-forties. The university had recently opened a state-of-the-art fitness center, pool and all, and it was free for faculty and students. I started walking. That's all I could do. Everything hurt, but I kept showing up day after day. One of the perks of being faculty is that you have flexibility with your schedule so there was time to walk, go home, and get ready for work.

I did everything I could to make my workouts more pleasurable in hopes of sustaining them. Technology wasn't quite what it is today. I used to work out on the elliptical machine using a portable CD player so I could listen to music, trying to hold it still so it wouldn't skip. (It always skipped.) Later that year, Eric gave me an iPod for my birthday and that changed everything. My workouts became a lot more enjoyable. I could download all the music I wanted, which made exercising a lot more fun. Frankly, I don't enjoy exercising that much. I never have, but I knew it was important, so I kept going. But that iPod, man, it was amazing! Game-changer.

I had settled into a consistent routine. My eating was healthier due to Mom and Eric also wanting to eat healthier, and I had lost about sixty pounds. I was in the gym one morning when one of my students approached me with one of the Army ROTC faculty. My student introduced us and then the sergeant asked me if I wanted to work out with the cadets every morning at physical training, or "PT."

"Why would I want to do that?" I asked.

He told me they'd been watching me, and they were impressed with my dedication and progress. I assume my student had said something. They offered to help me meet my health goals if I was interested. He added, "If you decide to join us, meet us at 5:50 a.m. in front of the ROTC building. Oh, and wear your bathing suit under your workout clothes, we're going to be in the pool."

"Thanks, I'll think about it."

I had absolutely no intention of taking them up on their offer. None. However, the more I thought about it, the more intrigued I was. So, ten minutes before six the next morning, I found myself out in front of the ROTC building wearing my bathing suit underneath my sweats. I had no idea what I was getting into.

I had lost sixty pounds, but I still had another sixty to go. I was definitely starting to feel better physically. I was eating healthier, and I could tell I was getting stronger. I thought maybe they could help me reach my health goals after all. What I wasn't prepared for was the officer leading PT that morning. He was all muscles with a too-tight T-shirt and a huge, bright white, toothy grin.

Oh, Lord, I thought. *What have I gotten into? How can I be in a bathing suit in front of this guy?*

He introduced himself, welcomed me, and explained what was going to happen. There were about twenty ROTC cadets who seemed cool with a professor hanging out with them. They were all very nice to me, but I was a nervous wreck.

We started with sit-ups, push-ups (modified for me), and some stretches. I couldn't do much, but I hung in there. Then we went to the pool. Now, I was scared. I'm not a good swimmer. I can do a bit of a sidestroke, but no one would confuse me with someone who could actually swim. I was doing my best to keep up (I couldn't). At some point, I found myself hanging on to the side of the pool for dear life. I was trying to catch my breath while everyone else was doing fireman carries the length of the pool. Each of the cadets alternated carrying someone the length of the pool and then they would switch. I couldn't even carry myself the length of the pool, let alone someone else.

One of the cadets swam over to me and said, "Ma'am, it's your turn."

"I think I'll just hang out here and watch."

"I understand, Ma'am. It's your turn."

One member of the cadre came over and suggested I figure out how to get myself down the length of the pool. They wouldn't make me carry anyone, but he explained that no one would be allowed to leave until I got to the other end of the pool.

I thought, *You are kidding me! You realize I'm not actually in the Army, right?!*

I could have said, "No."

I could have gotten out of the pool (or tried to, I was really tired) and left. But I found that I didn't want to let them or myself down.

I have no idea where I got the energy—much less the ability or the courage—but slowly and not very surely, I swam the length of that pool. My lungs were burning and my arms felt like dead weights, but I got to the other end. When I looked up, there they were. Every single cadet, waiting for me. No one had pity in their eyes, no one looked like they had anywhere else they needed to be. They weren't frustrated, impatient, or angry. They were just lined up waiting for me. It was incredibly powerful.

Afterwards, I was sitting on the bleachers and one member of the cadre came over and asked if I was okay. I had tears in my eyes. I said I was just a bit overwhelmed. I had never pushed myself that hard before and second, I had never experienced that level of support.

He nodded and said, "That's what we do. We don't abandon our team and, as of today, you're one of us. We will always wait for you."

I can't even begin to describe the impact of what he said to me. In that moment, I felt like I belonged to one of the greatest teams in existence. After that, I showed up every day at 5:50 a.m. for PT. Rain or shine.

I'd been working out with them for about six months when one of the cadre called me. "I'll be at the track tomorrow at 0600 for PT tests. I expect you to be there."

I reminded him, "You do realize, I don't actually have to take a PT test."

"You're one of us now. I'll see you in the morning."

I showed up, as he knew I would. I knew they didn't have to invest the energy in me. They didn't have to treat me as one of their own, but they did. They promised to help me reach my goals, and they were serious. The PT test started. No one expected me to qualify or pass the test, but I was expected to finish.

I expected me to finish.

Everyone started by running two miles. So, there I was, running, albeit very slowly, around the track. About a mile and a half in, I felt something give in the back of my knee. It was excruciatingly painful. I started walking and a cadet I didn't know ran up alongside me.

"You can do this, Dr. Norling. Just keep going."

Through clenched teeth I said, "I appreciate that, but I'm hurt. My leg."

He thought I needed encouragement so he kept saying, "You can make it, Dr. Norling. You can do this." He offered to run alongside me until I finished. No matter what I said, he wouldn't leave my side. I knew it wasn't smart when I did it, but I hobbled the rest of the way with this young cadet at my side. I don't even remember what my injury was (it was bad enough that the entire top half of my leg was severely bruised, and I had to stay off it for a while), but I will always remember that young cadet making sure I finished.

I had become a kind of mascot for the Army ROTC program, in a good way. I became good friends with the leadership and enjoyed getting to attend ROTC events. I was their biggest supporter on campus. At one point, they sent me to leadership training at Fort Lewis in Washington State to represent our university. While there, there was an opportunity to rappel a forty-foot wall. I jumped at the chance because a few months earlier, I learned how to rappel during ROTC exercises and enjoyed the challenge. I rocked that wall and asked to go again!

What I didn't realize at the time was that my experience with the Army ROTC was teaching me how to trust. Not only others but myself. It was rebuilding confidence in myself and increasing my self-worth, which had been beaten and battered over the years. I was pushing myself physically harder than I ever had, and I knew they had my back. What a gift that was. I was doing things I never thought I could do, and no one was prouder of me than they were.

They always waited for me. Every single time.

One morning after PT, I was sitting in the office talking with one member of the cadre.

Out of the blue he asked, "How would you like to jump out of an airplane?"

I was sure I misunderstood him. "What?"

He said the Golden Knights, the Army's demonstration and competition parachute team, was coming to the university, and they wanted me to tandem jump with them. I didn't know what to say. They were offering the opportunity to the university president, other senior leaders, and me. A lowly assistant professor.

"Why me?"

"Because you've earned it."

I had to think about it. In all my crazy adventures, nowhere on my bucket list was skydiving. Later, while I was talking with my mom and brother about it, I realized how much I really wanted to do this. I said yes. It was an incredible honor and, frankly, you don't get the opportunity to tandem jump with the Golden Knights every day. Of course, I was going to do it and then it occurred to me, there might be a weight restriction. Oh, hell.

I reached out to Lt. Col. Chris Speer, who led the ROTC program, and asked if there was a weight limit. He told me there was. I was crushed. I was twenty-one pounds above that, and they were coming in less than a month. I told him I weighed more than that but would like the chance to meet the weight limit.

He hesitated. "I'll hold your seat as long as I can. But whatever you do, do not endanger your health for this."

I agreed and he said he would check in with me the weekend before the jump.

Who knew I wanted to jump out of a plane so badly? Obviously, it was more than that, it was about proving something to myself. It was about facing fears and the exhilaration of doing something that few can say they did. I was talking with Eric about it, who had no clue why I would want to do such a thing.

"How bad do you want to do this?" he asked.

"Bad."

He had been a wrestler in school, so he put together a diet and exercise plan that included two-a-day workouts and a no-carb, insanely low-calorie diet. I lived on sugar-free popsicles to help curb the nausea, which I constantly had. I still can't eat sugar-free popsicles to this day.

A week later, one member of the cadre asked if he could sit in on one of my classes. I had no idea why, but I said sure. Toward the end of the class, he raised his hand and asked if he could say something. He announced to my class that I would be jumping with the Golden Knights. He also mentioned that I was going to need everyone's support to meet the requirements and told them I was doing two-a-day workouts. If they saw me in the gym, they were to cheer me on. For the next three weeks, whenever one of my students saw me working out, they made sure they gave me a high five.

Some of them would jump on the exercise equipment next to me even if they were done for the day. My entire class was showing up to help me reach my goals. Word got out to other staff and faculty, and they did the same thing when they saw me. It was incredible. I don't usually like that kind of attention, especially if it's related to my weight. Now it would be public knowledge whether I succeeded or not, whether I met my goal. I pushed that thought aside and embraced all of the encouragement and kept moving forward.

I was supposed to jump on a Monday. The Saturday before the jump, I got on the scale. I was two pounds below the limit! I had done it! With the help of my class, the support of my ROTC buddies, and Mom and Eric, I met the weight limit. Lt. Col. Speer called me Sunday night. I told him I reached my goal. He was incredibly proud of me.

"I'll see you on the ground," he said.

I was elated and proud and scared to death. What had I gotten myself into? I now had to jump out of a perfectly good airplane.

The next morning, I showed up at the hangar where we would meet the Golden Knights and prepare for the jump. I introduced myself to the president of the university and his senior leaders. I know he was trying to figure out why I was there. We met the Golden Knights parachute team and the partner we were assigned to tandem with, and they taught us how to land. Then we waited. And waited. And waited. We were in a weather delay. After a few hours, it was clear that the weather wasn't going to change, and the jump was canceled. I was so disappointed. I found out from my mom later that there were hundreds of people at the landing zone waiting for us. My students were all there, along with Mom and Eric and other faculty and students. While I didn't get to jump, I learned an important lesson about myself: I could do anything if I put my mind to it. I was stronger than I thought, and I had a support system unlike anything I had ever experienced.

Chapter Nine

A few years after we all moved to Pensacola, Mom started having health issues. At one point, she was in the ICU, and we weren't sure she was going to make it. I called her sisters to come down and down they came. That's something I appreciate about our family, if you needed them, they were there. No questions asked. Mom ended up pulling through, but having her sisters with her as she recuperated was the best medicine for her. It also gave Eric and me a little break. Whenever any of our family was in the hospital, we were always there by the bedside. We didn't trust anyone to take as good care of them as we could. It was exhausting, but we still did it. Every single time.

Mom's health kept getting worse, though. She found herself in and out of the hospital numerous times. I loved my mom fiercely. I never got tired of talking with her, and we spoke on the phone at least once a day since the day I became an adult and started living on my own. She was my heartbeat. My lifeline. When she would go into the hospital, she almost always ended up with mental encephalopathy, an infection that would make her confused. Her voice would take on a strange affect. When she spoke, she didn't make sense, and her eyes became dull. We could always tell when she was getting sick by the color of her eyes and the pitch of her voice. It was subtle, but we could tell, and we were never wrong. We'd take her to the emergency room because we knew what was about to happen. Most of the time, they didn't believe us, and we'd have to bring her back within six or eight hours. Then they would finally start treatment for the very thing that we told them was happening when we were there earlier. It was incredibly frustrating. No one would listen to us even though we knew exactly what was about to happen. Sometimes it would get so bad we'd have to call an ambulance. For the first few days, she wouldn't know we were even there.

I always knew she was going to be ok when I walked into her hospital room and she greeted me with "Hello, Daughter."

I'd always answer, "Hello, Mother." At that point, I could breathe again. Until the next time.

A few months later, Mom was sick again. She was hospitalized but they couldn't figure out what was going on. Mom was getting worse. Nothing anyone had done thus far was making a difference, and now she was unable to communicate at all, which scared us. We knew it scared Mom. I had to call in the palliative care team. I happened to know them, and they came right over. We were desperate for answers. We knew she felt trapped because she couldn't talk. We could see it in her eyes. Eric and I stayed by her side and were exhausted, but we were not going to leave her. Not for a second. The situation was getting worse, and I had reached my breaking point.

They moved her to a different floor, and suddenly I just couldn't go see her. I was frozen, unable to walk down that hallway. I'd never felt that way before. I just couldn't see her knowing she was so lost and scared. This was the only time I couldn't face something this hard, but I couldn't move.

Eric was sitting with me. I told him I couldn't do it. I couldn't go see Mom right now. He told me, "Gretch, I got this. Just rest for a while."

I watched him slowly get up out of the chair in the waiting room, all six-feet-three-inches of him, with his body battered from years of herniated disks and back surgeries. His left shoulder drooped like it always did, and with his uneven gait, he stood up as tall as I've ever seen him stand. He walked down that long hallway towards Mom. He stood with her for hours, holding her hand and talking to her. It was so hard for him to stand for any length of time, but he stood there. He wouldn't leave her. I know he must have been thinking of the time we nearly lost him as a kid, when he was hit by that truck. Mom wouldn't leave his side then, so he wouldn't leave her side now.

I finally pulled myself together and joined him. While we were standing there, Mom woke up.

She opened her eyes and took us in. "You found me. I was so lost, but you found me."

We were all crying, but Eric said, "Mom, we'll always find you."

Once we knew she was okay, we both went home and collapsed. That was the most difficult experience we'd ever had with Mom so far, but she was the center of our lives. We'd walk through fire for her, and we knew she'd do the same for us. I don't know what all the doctors did, but they pulled her out of it, and we brought her home.

A few months later, I met my husband, Ronn, on an online dating website. I'd been on the site earlier in the year but had let my subscription expire. In September, I received an email saying someone who I had had a few conversations with earlier in the year wanted to get a hold of me. I had to rejoin to get the message. The message that prompted me back to the website turned out to be nothing I wanted to pursue. But in that thirty-day timeframe of the extended subscription, I met Ronn. I don't care what anyone says, the universe makes things happen if you're paying attention. We were meant to be. I had no intention of rejoining the website, but here we are, married for fifteen years now.

He is the love of my life.

I remember when I knew he was the one. We had been dating for a week, and I was going to spend the weekend at his house, an hour away. We were on the phone so he could give me directions and make sure I got there safely. I remember to this day how even though I was only a mile or two away from his house, he stayed on the phone with me and was standing at the end of his driveway, on his phone, until he had me in his sights. I saw him standing there, phone in hand, making sure I arrived safely. I was in love. Knowing he would never, ever leave me hanging made my heart swell. The fact that he was the most handsome, kindest, smartest, generous, funny, and loving man I'd ever met, didn't hurt, either. I didn't have a chance.

Ronn's daughter, Branwyn, was in high school when we met. Like any normal sixteen-year-old, she wasn't particularly interested in her dad's new girlfriend. In fact, I'm pretty sure she had no interest in me at all. I couldn't blame her. I figured if Ronn and I got serious, we'd have plenty of time to get to know each other. Over time, we developed a very close relationship, and I love her dearly! She's truly a gift, and I'm blessed to have her as my daughter. She calls me Mom, which makes my heart smile.

About a year after Ronn and I got married, we moved to Memphis for my new job. Mom decided it was finally time to leave Pensacola and go home. She knew her health was declining, and she wanted to spend what time she had left with her sisters. Eric did not want to go; he loved Pensacola. He had a lot of friends, was playing music with a band he loved, and had made a life for himself. But where Mom went, Eric went, too. He was her primary caregiver; he took great care of her and vice versa. Ronn and I bought a small condo up there, so we'd have a place to stay when we visited. We just gave them the keys.

After they moved home, Mom continued to have episodes that would land her in the hospital. It was a delicate balance trying to keep her out of the hospital. Between infections, potassium spikes, kidney issues, and other health problems, it wasn't unusual for her to be in the hospital every few months. She was getting tired of it. She knew she was living on borrowed time and spoke frankly about it. The last time she had been in the hospital, they had intubated her. I was waiting outside the door while they were taking her off the ventilator. As soon as I entered her room, I knew she was angry.

"Don't you ever let them do that to me again."

And she meant it. We promised. No more ventilators. We hadn't made the decision to intubate her or not; we hadn't had the opportunity. The emergency room staff did it to save her life without asking, but she didn't care. She was mad.

I realized then and there how important it was to know how our loved ones wanted to be treated, especially when they have no voice. The worst time to have this conversation is when everyone is scared or having to make difficult decisions. At this point everyone is just guessing, and the situation is fraught with emotion. This is frequently when spouses, siblings, and children disagree about what should be done. There are a lot of excellent tools out there to guide these difficult conversations well before the time comes. *Five Wishes* is a document that provides families with a framework for identifying what each of us would like to happen should we not be able to speak for ourselves. Think about it: do you really want someone who is scared, anxious, overwhelmed, and often exhausted to have to guess at what you want done?

We were lucky that Mom had always made it very clear what she wanted. Sometimes we didn't have a say in the moment, but there was never guessing involved. We knew what Dad wanted, too. You'd be surprised how individualistic we all are in our preferences. We make a lot of assumptions in our lives, but carrying out our loved ones' last wishes should be based on their preferences, not ours. Even having formal documentation filled out doesn't guarantee that there won't be disagreements, but it does provide everyone, including the clinical staff, with important information on how to proceed.

Chapter Ten

A few years later, Ronn and I ended up in Eastern Kentucky for yet another new professional opportunity for me. While there, I received a phone call from one of Dad's neighbors. She told me he wasn't doing very well and something serious was going on. They had heard gunshots and were worried about him. I didn't know what I could do from Kentucky, so I called Eric and Mom, who lived about thirty minutes from Dad.

Not surprisingly, Eric and Dad had a complicated relationship. Dad had a complicated relationship with everyone, but it was most complicated with Eric. Eric had legitimate reasons for his anger, but no matter how mad he was at Dad, if Dad needed something, Eric did his best to help him, even if it caused him great pain. Mom was the same. So was I.

Eric called Dad and didn't get an answer, so he and Mom jumped in the car and drove to his house. They couldn't get near the house because the police were already there. There was an ambulance standing by. Eric called me and stayed on the phone with me while they tried to figure out what was going on. It was in the evening and the house was dark. He had had his power turned off earlier that day due to nonpayment. This wasn't unusual, but the gunshots were. He hadn't had a drink in many years, but he abused pills, and we assumed he was out of his supply. Over the years, even after he got sober, it became clear Dad had some serious mental and emotional issues that had never been addressed. His alcoholism had overshadowed it for a long time. He wasn't a bad guy, but he wasn't well most of the time. He had stretches of his life when he did really well, like when he was in Alcoholics Anonymous or following treatment, but as is often the case, an addict gets one thing under control and replaces the addiction with something else. Dad's something else was pills.

It was dark now and they couldn't see anything, but they could hear the gunshots and so could I. The police kept Mom and Eric informed about what was going on and then they would tell me. Every time we'd hear a gunshot, we expected them to bring Dad out in a body bag.

It's hard to describe what was going through my mind on the other end of that phone. I was petrified that he would be shot by the police. My dad was never one to back down from a fight. My heart was beating so hard, I could hear it in my ears. I stayed on the phone with Mom and Eric throughout the entire situation. I don't know who was calming whom down more. Mom and Eric seemed to be handling it better than I was, which wasn't surprising. I think it was harder to be on the end of the phone feeling helpless. At least we could support each other. Eric always handled events around Dad with great strength, even considering all the drama and Dad's bad behavior over the years. I didn't want him to die, especially like that.

After an hour or so, the police got into the house, and they took Dad away in an ambulance. Dad wasn't shooting at anyone, nor was he intending to harm himself. He was having some kind of psychotic episode. They finally informed Eric and Mom that he was unharmed, and they were taking him to the emergency room. They followed. Eric went into the back where he was being treated.

From what Eric reported to us later, Dad was out of his mind. He was yelling and fighting everyone. Dad was not a big man, and he was in his seventies by then, but he was still strong. It took Eric, the big man that he was, and three other men, including law enforcement, to restrain Dad enough to administer a shot to calm him down. They transferred him to a larger hospital in Saginaw. I was on my way to Michigan the next day. I wasn't able to talk with Dad yet, so I had to trust the doctors that they would take good care of him. I was never confident that they would.

He was obviously in pain, physically, mentally, and emotionally. I sometimes wondered how Dad felt throughout this. Was he scared? I'd never known my dad to be scared, but I'm sure he was many times. I have no way of knowing because we never talked about it afterward. Everyone was traumatized by this. I don't know if he was out of his mind on pills or if he was out of pills and fully cognizant. If he recalled any of it, he never said anything. I prefer to think he didn't remember any of it. We sure did, though.

I don't want anyone to think there weren't good, fun, loving days with Dad. We had a lot of them. It's just that I seem to remember the hard days more. When I was in my early twenties, I was living in Atlanta and had come home for a visit. Dad and I went fishing, just the two of us. It was a perfect day. I don't even remember if we caught any fish, but we were so comfortable just being together, talking and laughing. When I got back to Atlanta, Dad sent me a card saying how much fun it was and just watching the joy on my face meant the world to him. Dad didn't send cards very often so when he did, it meant a lot.

A few years later, I moved to Utah to work at a ski resort. I moved frequently, ever the wanderer. I guess I was searching for something, probably myself. Moving to a new environment seemed to be how I thought I'd accomplish that. I don't think it worked, but I sure had a lot of fun. One year, Dad came to visit me by himself. We had a ball. Just the two of us exploring. At one point, we found ourselves on a road that was so treacherous that I wasn't sure we'd survive. I was driving and there was no place to pull over and switch drivers. Dad was so calm and confident in my ability to get us through to safer ground. I, on the other hand, was a nervous wreck. I was white-knuckling the steering wheel, not daring to look down at the ravine. Dad was talking as though we were on a Sunday drive in the country. I wish I had had that much confidence in myself back then.

Dad's health started deteriorating rapidly following the mental breakdown. At one point, we thought he only had a few days left with him, so we called the family to the hospital. He had some serious conversations during that time. He told Eric how proud he was of him. They had started to heal their relationship a bit, and I know that meant a lot to both of them. The person he most wanted to see, though, was Mom. Always Mom. Even though they had been divorced for years, she came. Her health wasn't great, either, but she came to the hospital. I watched her walk down the corridor, alone, using her cane in that crooked way she walked, to say her goodbyes. You can say a lot about my dad, but he loved my mom. It wasn't necessarily a healthy love, but it was deep. They'd been together since she was fourteen and had been married for thirty-five years before they divorced.

The nurse told me later that Dad's face lit up when she walked into the room. It was obvious how much he loved her. I don't know all he said, but I know my mom was gracious as always and told him she loved him, too. And she did. During our visit, I was visibly upset, and Dad hated it when I cried. He tended to get annoyed. He told me he was proud of me, but I always knew he was. He said he loved me. I don't know that we had a lot left to say to each other. Of all of us, I probably had the best relationship with Dad but that wasn't saying a lot. Loving Dad wasn't ever easy, but we still all showed up for him when he needed us. When he didn't need us, he didn't really want us around that much which was fine by us.

Dad held on and got well enough to go into an assisted living facility. He didn't want to go. He'd lived on his own for a long time and wanted to go home. He couldn't, though. His house wasn't inhabitable, and he needed ongoing care. After a few weeks he settled in and started to thrive. I would check in regularly with the nurse, and once she told me that Dad had been dancing the day before with some of the nurses. Some musicians had come in to play and he found a partner to dance with. He was always a fantastic dancer. It put a big smile on my face to hear that he felt good enough to dance.

A few weeks later, I got a call from the facility. They had gone into Dad's room, and he was on the floor. They called for an ambulance. He immediately went into surgery where they found a hole in his stomach lining. All his food and medication had been going directly into his body. The doctor called me. He said Dad was in bad shape and that I should come home. They transferred him to Saginaw for more intensive care. The doctor said he probably wouldn't make it for long and I should get to Saginaw if I wanted to say goodbye.

We were still living in Eastern Kentucky, so it was only about an eight-hour drive to get there. The problem was the snow and ice storm that was hitting Ohio and Michigan. I got on the road and prayed I'd get there in time. Mom and Eric would meet me there. Ronn would come later.

The angels were with me during that drive. There was ice everywhere. Cars were in ditches and accidents were happening all around me. My car had ice all over it, except for the windshield. I have no idea how that was even possible, but I made it without any problems. I walked onto his floor and his medical team met me at the elevator. They wanted to update me on his condition. He didn't have long and while they had mentioned intubation to Dad, it really wasn't an option. It would just be painful and prolong the inevitable. They recommended hospice care. I asked if they had explained all of this to Dad, and they said they were waiting for me. Dad was fully cognizant. He understood everything that was going on. When I walked in, I kissed him on the forehead and held his hand. He wasn't a particularly demonstrative man, but he was glad I was there. He asked me about having a tube put down his throat and I explained that it wasn't an option now. It would just be painful and uncomfortable and wouldn't help.

He looked at me and said, "Am I checking out, now?"

"Yeah, Dad. I'm sorry." It was all I could say.

Eric walked in at that point and the two of us just sat with him. At some point, Dad looked at Eric and said, "Make sure I'm comfortable."

Eric knew what he was asking and promised he would. I left the two of them alone. I knew Dad had some things he wanted to say to Eric. He came out a few minutes later with tears in his eyes. We met with the medical team and requested comfort care. It was too late for hospice. Eric kept his promise and Dad was made comfortable.

I left to check into the hotel where Mom and Eric were staying. Even in her failing health, Mom was our rock. She didn't go see Dad again. She didn't need to. Eric and I went back and sat with Dad. We held his hands. At some point, he lifted off his oxygen mask.

"Don't be afraid," he told me.

Through my tears, I said, "I love you, Dad."

He passed shortly after with both Eric and me by his side.

We planned his funeral and held it a few days later at the funeral home. He looked a lot older than his seventy-three years. Funerals are always hard, and Dad's was no different. He was finally free and out of pain. He had lived a hard life, much of his own doing, but he was loved. Mom was there and she said nothing but nice things about him. No one would have expected anything different. She was always conflicted, though. She loved Dad deeply, but she didn't like him anymore. He had caused her great pain, but we know she forgave him because that's how she lived her life.

Dad was cremated, and before we had a chance to inter his ashes, we lost Mom, too.

The last time I spoke to Mom was on a Thursday, about six months later. We spoke pretty much every day, even if it was only for a few minutes. It was a short conversation; she was tired and resting. She had just gotten out of the hospital again and was trying to get her strength back. Each hospitalization just kept taking more and more out of her. I had changed jobs again, and we were living in Miami. Ronn was working in Mississippi on an assignment, so we were in two different places for the time being. I knew if something was wrong, Eric would call me. It had been an ongoing conversation our entire lives. At first it was Chris's health and then it was either Dad's or Mom's health issues or his, or mine, for that matter. I felt like that's all we ever talked about, though I know that's not true.

The following Saturday morning, I didn't want to get out of bed. I'm normally an early riser, but I just wanted to stay in bed. I couldn't explain why, I just felt lethargic and sad. I finally got out of bed mid-morning and my phone was full of messages from Eric and Ronn. Mom had died in her sleep. The medical examiner said it was from natural causes. Eric was in shock. I can't even imagine what he was going through, waking up to find Mom had died. I immediately started making arrangements to get home. I had little time to do it but managed to get a flight into Detroit where I'd meet Ronn, and we would drive to Midland.

I was beside myself. I couldn't think. I didn't know what to pack. I couldn't seem to make a decision, and I couldn't stop crying. When I got to the Miami airport, I could barely speak at all. People were asking me if I was ok, and I'd just shake my head. Everyone could tell something serious had happened. Strangers were kind and offered me tissues and water. When I got on the plane, I finally closed my eyes, but I was still crying. One of the passengers wanted me to change seats with her so she could sit with her husband. I shook my head, no. Just, no.

I got to Detroit late and caught up with Ronn and we drove the ninety minutes to Midland. We were exhausted, but I had to see Eric who was waiting at the hotel for us. When I saw him, I just hugged him. Hard. I knew we'd get through this, but it was going to be brutal. We had a lot to do, but first, we all had to get some rest.

We could have lost Mom so many times before we actually did. Because we were all so close, there was nothing left unsaid. We weren't shy about saying, "I love you," every time we spoke or saw each other. Luckily, Mom was very direct in talking about what she wanted done at her funeral, so we knew what to do.

After she had gotten extremely sick in Pensacola, she started talking more and more about what she wanted when that day came. I remember helping her make her bed one day when she brought it up. I immediately started to tear up. She said she had to talk to me because she couldn't talk to Eric about it. I understood, and with tears in my eyes, I listened to Mom tell me everything she needed to tell me. Mom never shied away from hard conversations. She was very matter-of-fact about these things.

I had come home for her seventy-fifth birthday and ended up taking her to a doctor's appointment. We stopped at Taco Bell on the way home. She was talking about life after she was gone. She knew her time on earth was limited and needed to talk about some things. As usual, I got teary. She asked me why I was getting so sad. I told her I was going to miss her terribly.

"Oh Gretchen," she said, "but we have so many memories. I'll always be with you." The memory of that moment still makes me tear up. But, as usual, Mom was right. She's always with me. After she died, Mom came to me in a dream and I swear, I felt her hug me. I really did.

Mom had a Catholic funeral. It's what she wanted, and it was beautiful. All of her friends and family were there. She was so loved. She was a light for so many, and I don't think she really knew that. She had a way of making everyone feel like they were the most special person in the world to her because they were. Mom's gift was seeing people as they were, accepting them fully, and then loving them unconditionally. Did she ever feel worthy of all the love she got? I think so. Did she ever forgive herself for not leaving Dad for good earlier? No.

I knew Eric was going to have an especially difficult time when Mom died. I stayed as long as I could before going back to Miami, but at some point, I had to go back to work. I was really worried about him, though. I had promised Mom that I'd always make sure he was ok and that's what I intended to do. Eric was lost without Mom and so was I. I knew that Mom had been preparing us for the last few years to go on without her. She would be furious if she knew we stayed in a sad place too long and didn't continue to grab onto all of the joy and happiness still to come. If Mom taught us anything, she taught us how to embrace life no matter how hard it got. Her answer to everything was to love unconditionally and to nurture happiness everywhere you could, especially in places where it was hard to find. Especially in those places. As long as we were together, we were happy.

I think that's why Mom loved dandelions, because they grew in spite of their conditions and brought light to the world with their bright yellow color. At the first sign of spring, up came the dandelions no matter how brutal the winter, and she loved seeing those little yellow miracles, little pops of yellow everywhere. They made her smile. Dandelions became especially important to me when she died. I incorporated them into my logo for my podcast and website. Dandelions remind me of my mom, and I smile every time I see one. I even wear a dandelion pin. Mom had always brought us great comfort; she was our rock. Now, Eric and I would have to do that for each other.

Unfortunately, Eric's health wasn't very good. His diabetes wasn't under control, and he was now going to be alone, and I didn't like that. His back was getting worse, and his healthcare was getting more challenging. Pain control in our country is shameful. There was always a battle around pain medication. He spent a considerable amount of time in bed because the pain was so bad he couldn't stand or sit for very long. We talked every day except when he ran out of pain medicine. When he ran out of his meds, I wouldn't hear from him for a few days. He didn't want me to know what he was going through. I can't even imagine what that experience was like for him. He was on high doses of extremely strong narcotics, but his tolerance was so high that nothing much helped. He suffered a lot and in silence. I couldn't do anything to help him. It broke my heart.

Chapter Eleven

Miami was yet another new city, a new professional opportunity, and another chance to reinvent myself. Since Ronn was working in Mississippi, I was there by myself most of the time. We found a new, gated apartment complex that had a lot of amenities, including a gym. As I had done many times before, I decided I would start fresh and try and lose weight yet again. I knew what foods I should be eating for the most part, but never quite integrated the exercise piece long-term. I've always found that people who are overweight know a lot about how to lose weight, we just have difficulty putting it into practice. In my case, it wasn't sustainable. Like every time before, I thought, *This is going to be it! I'm going to make it happen!* I started walking at a local park on the weekends (even though it was way too hot to be doing that), visited the local farmer's markets to buy the fresh fruits and vegetables I knew I needed, and every morning before work, I'd workout at the apartment gym.

It lasted for a few months, long enough to start seeing a difference. I felt encouraged and powerful. I thought maybe I'd figured it out. I had some momentum going and I thought, *Boy was Ronn going to be excited when he saw me next!* Although he had never said a word about my weight and always loved me unconditionally, I felt self-conscious at such a high weight. A few months later, I started having irregular and extremely heavy periods. I had never quite made it to the other side of menopause, but I knew this wasn't right. The bleeding would come and go so at first, I didn't think much of it. After about six months, I mentioned it to my primary care doctor, but he didn't pursue it, so I just dealt with it. He, unsurprisingly, attributed it to my obesity and never ordered any additional tests. I was told to lose weight. Given that was always the response to any medical issue I had, I started to believe it, too. I let it go.

The bleeding continued over the next few years. It made it difficult to work out, but it shouldn't have made any difference in how I ate. As was often the case, after about six months, I stopped eating nutritious foods, my portion size grew, and working out came to a halt. It happens gradually. Instead of working out daily, I'd begin skipping days. Instead of preparing my meals, I would eat out more. After a while, I had fully returned to my unhealthy habits. My weight came back, as it always did, and then some. This is the pattern I'd been following my entire life. I was so disappointed in myself, although not surprised. My confidence was shot, and I started to become depressed.

I would go years between weight loss attempts. I'd beat myself up so badly for not having any willpower that it would take years to get the courage to try again.

I'd like to eliminate the word willpower. I hate that word. It sets us up to fail every time.

What I would finally figure out is that it has nothing to do with willpower and everything to do with setting up a process and infrastructure that would support my goals. It would have nothing to do with how I was feeling in the moment or that day. Once I figured that out, I found freedom.

A few years later, having moved to North Georgia for yet

another job, I found myself bleeding so heavily that I had to put towels and pads on our bed at night because I would bleed through everything. One day, I was bleeding so heavily at work that the bathroom looked like a crime scene. There was blood everywhere. Sitting on the toilet, I could feel the blood clots falling out of me. Some were the size of golf balls. I cleaned it up the best I could and called Ronn. He met me at the emergency room.

The emergency room was packed. I sat there with my husband for hours, bleeding and changing out sanitary pads and tampons every thirty minutes. Huge blood clots were coming out of my body, and I was scared. I was also exhausted. I'm sure I was losing a lot of blood. At some point, the bleeding stopped. I asked the person at the front desk if they had any idea how long it would be, and they said at least another 6-8 hours, so we went home.

During my lifetime, I have spent a significant amount of time navigating the healthcare system for either myself or one of my family members. Rarely did it go well. One memorable experience happened around the time I was first diagnosed with thyroid cancer while I was living in New York. I had found myself with a painful Bartholin cyst. I had never felt pain like that before. Because they form on the outer lobes of the vagina, it becomes difficult to sit or stand. In fact, gravity is not your friend in this situation, because when I stood up, the pain was the absolute worst. I was in tears. They're common in young women, especially those who have never had children. They are usually not painful, but mine was excruciating, and it was unusually large. I went to the emergency room because I couldn't stand the pain any longer. I was on a gurney in the hallway because they didn't have any rooms in the back. It was a busy hospital, and some of the patients were prisoners. I was by myself and incredibly uncomfortable, not being able to sit or stand without severe pain, and I was stuck in the open where periodically someone would come by and as discreetly as they could, examine me. I remember lying there next to a prisoner who was handcuffed to his bed with a police officer guarding him. I would have been more nervous, but by then, they had given me strong pain medication, so I was a little more relaxed than normal. Ultimately, they admitted me, and surgery was scheduled for the next morning.

I was in my room, waiting to get prepped for surgery, when the medical team was making their rounds. There were multiple resident doctors and medical students on the team and the attending physician wanted each one of them to see my cyst. In fact, he wanted all of them to see it because apparently it was "huge," so they lifted the sheet to take a look. At least they asked permission, but it was as embarrassing as you can probably imagine. One of the residents decided he needed to examine me. He pressed on the cyst, and I cried out in pain, but he kept examining me.

Finally, I yelled, "Stop!! Get out of my room!" I was furious. A few minutes later, the nurse came in to prepare me for surgery, and I never saw them again. Just before they took me back, I called my professors to tell them I was on my way to surgery, but I would be in class on Monday and would make up all of my work. At least that's what I think I said, I was pretty loopy. They probably wondered why I was calling them at all.

From a lifetime of experience talking to doctors, I knew I had to advocate for myself and keep doing it until I got real help. After Ronn and I got home from our Emergency Room trip, I called my primary care physician, and she got me in to see an OB/GYN the next day. He immediately put me on progesterone to regulate the bleeding. He also ordered a vaginal ultrasound and did a biopsy. The ultrasound didn't pick anything up and the biopsy came back negative. I was relieved. The progesterone worked immediately and for the first time in over five years, the bleeding had stopped. I was fifty-seven years old, and we all knew I shouldn't be bleeding like that, but there was no further treatment planned. We were just going to monitor it.

I find two things interesting here. One, once again, a physician decided not to be aggressive and only monitor the situation. The same thing happened when I had thyroid cancer the first time.

There was no urgency, no rush to find out what was really going on even then, and now, I had been practically hemorrhaging, and he was just going to watch it. A few of my friends were going through a similar situation (it's not uncommon for women in their fifties) and for every single one of them, their physicians treated their symptoms aggressively by scheduling a hysterectomy immediately. No "monitoring," no "Let's wait and see what happens." Same symptoms, same excessive bleeding, large blood clots, and the same age. Completely different treatments. The only difference seemed to be that I was obese, and they weren't.

The bleeding remained at bay for almost a year. I was so grateful. I got my life back and we could go out if we wanted to or eat dinner with friends. I hadn't fully understood how much I was altering my life to accommodate the bleeding. I had regular checkups, but nothing appeared problematic. A year later, I started bleeding again. It was March 2020, and Covid had just started to emerge in the United States. I had accepted a new job in Mississippi and, with travel papers in hand, we moved to Gulfport. I had to find a new primary care doctor and lucked out when I met Dr. Jimmy Dimitriades. He was the program director for the family medicine residency we were starting. I asked around, wanting to find out if he was approachable and easy to talk to. Everybody raved about what a great doctor he was, so I asked him to be my doctor.

During our first appointment, I mentioned the bleeding and he jumped on it. He didn't think it was caused by my weight, or at least he was considering other explanations. He sent me to an OB/GYN who scheduled a D&C immediately. The sample was sent to the hospital pathology lab for evaluation. The results were mixed. Overall, the report said they thought I was okay but there were a few suspicious cells, so they wanted to send it to a university pathology lab. A few weeks later, I went back to see my OB/GYN for my results. He told me I had endometrial cancer, Stage 1A.

Not again, I thought. *Who gets cancer three times?*

I knew something wasn't right, but I had had numerous tests and biopsies, and everything had come back negative. The doctor who gave me the news was very kind. He said I would need to see a gynecological oncologist, and I had my choice of going to Ochsner in New Orleans or the Mitchell Cancer Institute at the University of South Alabama in Mobile. I chose USA. I thanked him and went back to the office. The doctor's office was across the street from the hospital where I worked. As I was walking back to my office, the news really started to register. I had cancer. Again.

I needed to go home. I didn't want to cry at work, and I knew I was on the verge. I told my coordinator what was going on, that I'd just been diagnosed with cancer, and that I was leaving for the day. I went straight home. Ronn was working in the yard. I got out of the truck and walked over to him. I told him it was cancer and started to cry. He just held me until I was ready to go inside.

I got an appointment with Dr. Jennifer Young Pierce, a gynecological oncologist and surgeon, relatively quickly. I immediately liked her. She would be doing my surgery and would be responsible for my follow-up care until I was in the clear. I was nervous. I was in poor physical health. I was still morbidly obese, had high blood pressure, and was prediabetic. I had to have the surgery; the tumor had to come out.

I knew I had to tell Eric. I had screwed this up twice before, so I called him as soon as I knew what we were doing and let him know. I told him I would have to have a radical hysterectomy, but I assured him I was going to be ok. I didn't know yet if I would have to have any additional treatment but would let him know once I did. I think he believed me. If he didn't, I wouldn't have blamed him. I stayed in very close contact with him throughout the process and made sure Ronn called him the second he knew I was safely out of surgery and what the prognosis was.

During my surgery, things got complicated. They had to stop because my heart rate dropped too low. I found out later it dropped to 28 bpm. A normal heart rate is 60-100 bpm for women. Elite athletes are known to have low resting heart rates, but I am not an elite athlete by any stretch. Unbeknownst to any of us, I had underlying bradycardia (a low heart rate). It's something else I need to watch, so I bought a wrist monitor. I've noticed that it's not unusual to have it drop to 46 bpm if I'm sitting quietly. I've been evaluated and have worn a heart monitor. So far, I'm okay.

The tumor was quite large, long and narrow, but not deep. It hadn't spread beyond my uterus. Dr. Pierce said she had a tough time due to my enlarged uterus. She wanted to remove it intact rather than cut it out in pieces since this would help prevent the spread of cancer cells. That too, was an ordeal, but she did it. It came out intact. While regular follow-up appointments would be required, no additional treatment was needed. I had been spared again.

Ronn was the most amazing partner to go through this experience with. I'd been through cancer before, but this was the first time he had gone through it with me. He was incredibly supportive and strong. He was at every appointment, asked important questions that I didn't remember to ask, and reassured me when I was scared. After the surgery, he never left my side until I told him to go home and get some rest. I had to stay in the hospital for a day or two and I know how exhausting it is to stand watch over someone you love. If you want to know how strong your marriage is, get a radical hysterectomy. The recovery is painful, it's embarrassing, and it's awkward. I was weak and in pain. I couldn't do anything for myself, at least for the first three or four days. If I wanted to sit down or get up from a chair, Ronn had to help me. We figured out how to best help me move without causing pain. It wasn't pretty but it worked. If I had to go to the bathroom, he had to help me. I couldn't sit down or get up from the toilet by myself. I couldn't even get dressed by myself. You know you've got a great partner when they're helping you put on clean underwear, and somehow make you laugh while you're doing it. It hurt to laugh, but it was healing. That's powerful.

During my first follow-up appointment with Dr. Pierce, she said, "Now we have to talk about what it means to be a cancer survivor. How to take care of yourself so you can live a healthy life."

She knew I had already survived cancer twice and probably knew all about this, but she wanted to have that conversation, anyway. We needed to talk about my weight. I needed to hear it, and she was right, I had to do something. I was weak from the surgery and my overall health was not good. So, did I do anything to improve my health right away? Nope.

Chapter Twelve

In February 2021, seven months after my radical hysterectomy, I was diagnosed with diabetes. I had gone in for a regular check-up and lab work. My A1c (blood glucose) was 6.7. I was officially diabetic. I had been prediabetic for years and had had plenty of opportunities to make healthy behavior changes, but I didn't. I wish everyone who is diagnosed prediabetic would take advantage of that diagnosis by making behavioral changes then and there to prevent full-blown diabetes, but most don't. Neither did I.

Dr. Dimitriades sat down across from me and said, "We need to have the talk, young lady. We need to get your weight down. What do you want to do? I want you to know, I'm here for you."

I knew what I needed to do. I told him, "Don't worry. I know what to do."

That night, I joined Weight Watchers for the third time. However, it would be a very different experience this time around.

I had been watching Eric fight complications of diabetes for the past ten years. His kidneys had already failed, and he was on dialysis. Dialysis is an amazing medical treatment for end-stage kidney disease. It can keep you alive for years, even decades, but it is terribly hard on your body, and it was taking its toll on Eric's. A blister on his foot had become infected and he fought the infection for almost two years before he had to have his leg amputated from below the knee. Now he had an infection in his other foot that wouldn't heal. His diabetes hadn't been fully controlled in years and it was ravaging his body. He'd been in a physical rehabilitation and assisted living facility for two years trying to get healthy enough to live independently again. He was only fifty-two and should have been enjoying his life, but his body wouldn't let him. It was heartbreaking, but he was always so optimistic. He was waiting for his prosthetic leg so he could be mobile enough to travel and come live near us. I'd been trying to figure out a way to make that happen for five years, ever since Mom died. It was a situation complicated by the fact that it took his losing his leg before he could even get disability. He'd been unable to work for a few years due to his back and now, after trying for almost ten years, he finally was approved for disability.

Ultimately, he never made it down to live near us, and that is my biggest regret in life. I didn't do enough to make it happen. It's all he wanted, to be with Ronn and me, but I just couldn't make it happen. It still keeps me up at night. I cry about it often.

Eric and I talked a lot. Sometimes, we talked several times a day. We'd talk about diabetes and what he wished he would have done differently when he was diagnosed in his mid-forties. He accepted responsibility for his part in his current situation. He knew he had let it get out of control and now it was too late to turn it around. The best he could do was spend whatever time he had with me. Given that we had already lost Mom, Dad, and Chris, it was now just the two of us and we were close. Really close. I flew home practically every time he was in the hospital, especially if it was serious, which it frequently was. If I wasn't there, I was on the phone with his doctors and nurses constantly. I did the same thing when Mom or Dad was in the hospital. I always felt it was never enough, though. I hated being so far away, but I never could find a well-paying job in or around my hometown or State. I tried for decades.

Looking back, I have spent most of my life navigating serious health issues, whether my own or my family's. Throughout my life, I would wake up in the middle of the night to make sure Chris was breathing when he was sick, or that Eric was okay because I knew he took such high doses of narcotics. I'd wake up to check my phone to see if there were phone calls from the hospital or the facility where Eric was to find out he was transported to the emergency room by ambulance. Sometimes, Eric would call and give me the news. Either way, I was always on the phone with doctors and nurses trying to find out what was going on and providing as much information as I could. I was a walking encyclopedia when it came to Mom's, Dad's, or Eric's past medical history.

When I heard the news that I was diabetic, I was scared but not surprised. Sooner than later, I was going to cross that line. Further, I knew my path would be similar to Eric's, there was no reason it wouldn't be. Even if you actively control your diabetes, most end up with serious complications from the disease, including limb amputations, losing your sight, and experiencing painful neuropathy, among other issues, and I already had the neuropathy. Plus, my office window overlooked our wound care center parking lot where I saw younger and younger people in wheelchairs or crutches, and morbidly obese people with missing limbs trying to get around. It was a daily reminder of my future. Finally, I didn't want Ronn, Branwyn, or her family to have to watch me deteriorate and become more and more dependent. I couldn't do that to them, especially if it was something I could prevent. Whatever I had control over, I had to make the changes, and I had to start now. I was already on blood pressure and pain medication and had been for years. I was taking Metformin to address my prediabetes and my

A1c was climbing. Plus, I didn't feel good, everything hurt. I was terribly unhealthy. I knew what the trajectory of my health was. I had to stop it. My life depended on it.

I had a full-on light bulb moment when I was told I was diabetic. I was driving home from work when I realized that I still had time. I still had time to make the changes necessary to become healthy so that I could prevent diabetes from destroying my body and my quality of life. After all, I had just been diagnosed diabetic that day. Three months ago, I was prediabetic. It dawned on me that I was one of the lucky ones. That hit me hard. Really hard.

I had time and my brother did not. Once I realized that, gratitude quickly followed. I felt a physical sensation all over my body when that realization hit. The best way to describe it was like a warming sensation. It was that strong of an epiphany. I had been given the gift of time! My diabetes wasn't so uncontrollable that it was ravaging my body like it had my brother's. I was grateful I had the resources to join a weight loss program. I could afford to buy healthy foods. Sometimes, eating healthily can be more expensive, but I didn't have to worry about buying groceries. Finally, I was grateful I had the support of my husband and my daughter.

Going to the doctor when you are morbidly obese is uncomfortable and causes a lot of anxiety for many of us. It always did for me. It goes beyond white coat syndrome, though. It had become what I felt, a dismissiveness and lack of respect for me as a person due to my obesity. Certainly, I had experienced compassionate physicians before, but it was rare. For the most part, going to the doctor wasn't a positive experience. I never felt heard, nor had I ever felt like they were glad I came in. Usually, I felt like they couldn't wait to get me out of their offices because dealing with obese patients, who can't or won't make the necessary behavior changes to get healthy, had to be frustrating. I felt like most had given up before they even got to know me. Maybe I had given up, too.

I liked one family medicine physician a lot. The first time I met him, he walked into the room and said, "Other than being under tall, what brings you in today?"

I thought that was quite funny and started to laugh. Great first impression! At least it made me open to what he had to say. I didn't immediately shut down and that was something. He did his best to actually help me, and I made some progress while going to him. Admittedly, humor can be tricky, but it works better with me than moral indignation and disdain. I'm just saying. Some physicians seem to think we can't tell how they feel about us. That's not true at all. We know.

Like many obese or morbidly obese patients, I typically avoided going to the doctor until I couldn't put it off any longer. No matter what I presented with, the visit became about my weight.

Earache? Lose weight. The flu? You weigh too much. UTI? It's because you're fat. Sprained wrist? Yep, if you weren't so heavy... they always brought it up and it was never productive.

They had no intention of helping me do anything about it. I know it's the most obvious health issue, and they feel obligated to talk about it, but it was never a conversation where they asked questions. It was always just negative or humiliating comments, and it never helped. Trust me, those of us who are overweight or obese are aware. We can see ourselves. Plus, strangers never hesitate to let us know how disgusted they are by our very existence. We know what size we wear and are depressed every time that size goes up.

The sad part is that there were so many missed opportunities to have a real conversation about why I was so unhealthy. Obviously, I ate too much but no one ever asked why, nor did anyone offer to run tests beyond my thyroid bloodwork to see if there was anything else going on. Was there a hormone imbalance? Who knows? What about other conditions that might contribute to my health problems? They were never interested in finding out. It was simple, I was just morbidly obese because I ate too much and moved too little. The end. Apparently, that explained everything. It wasn't until I was in my late forties that I even learned I had an autoimmune disease. I had no clue.

A lot of assumptions are made about obese patients. Research clearly shows that there is a significant weight bias in healthcare. The professionals who we must trust when we seek healthcare have been shown to have strong negative attitudes toward obese patients. Even those who specialize in obesity treatment can hold these biases. I have had doctors who actually thought I sat around eating entire pizzas or whole pans of lasagna and just sat on my couch watching television. An endocrinologist said that to my face during an office visit. This wasn't true, at all. I spent many winters skiing, even tackling expert black diamond trails (when I was in my late twenties). I was on a women's basketball team as a young woman and did my best to stay relatively active even if it hurt. And it always hurt.

I joined gyms over the years, but I never felt comfortable or welcomed there. Other members made that very clear. The looks, the stares, the eye rolls, and the cruel comments were enough to make it uncomfortable enough for me to stop going. I knew I wasn't welcome there. I often thought, *If people were really that concerned about my health, then they should have thrown me a parade, replete with balloons and a marching band, when I walked through the doors of a gym.* But no, that was not the case. There are more welcoming fitness centers today, and I hope that will make a difference for many.

I was sure things would be different this time. First, I felt Dr. Dimitriades was really my partner and advocate. There was no judgment, no condescending tone. He just sat down with me, and we talked. It was an actual conversation, not a lecture. He wasn't standing over me, and he didn't yell at me. He asked how he could help me, and I will always be appreciative of that.

"We'll do this together," he said. "We're partners in this."

No other physician had ever approached it that way, except for Dr. Pierce, after my hysterectomy. She, too, sat down with me and had the same conversation. No judgment. No condescension, just someone who was concerned and wanted to be my partner to help me succeed. She made recommendations, as well, and talked about tools that might be helpful. I just wasn't ready, yet. I was still reeling from having cancer a third time. Two compassionate physicians, six months apart, talking with me about my health, not at me, with me. I had never felt less judged. As I've said, I believe God puts people in my life to help me move forward in my journey at the right time and these two extraordinary physicians were doing just that. There were no two physicians more excited about my success. They celebrated right along with me. They still do.

Physicians talk with their patients about chronic disease management all the time, this is especially true for primary care doctors. Conversations about diabetes, heart disease, high blood pressure, high cholesterol, and other chronic conditions that require patient behavior change are held daily. It has to be a constant source of frustration for physicians who have these conversations without any results but it's incredibly frustrating for patients, too. Ultimately, the behavior change is up to the patient, but most of the time, it's a one-way conversation. Up until now, I rarely walked out of the exam room with any additional information or tools. For the record, I knew I was fat when I walked into the room. What I didn't know was how to fix it. Behavior change doesn't occur because we're given tons of information. It's more complicated than that. It's a missed opportunity between physicians and patients when the conversations aren't supportive or if they don't provide resources or tools to help patients begin their journey toward creating a healthier lifestyle. Telling patients that they need to "eat less and move more" isn't helpful. Whenever I was told that, I heard, *Good luck! You're on your own. We've given up on you.*

I didn't mention that I had joined Weight Watchers to my husband until a few days later. It's a bad habit I have, making decisions that affect other people and not telling them. At any rate, he was incredibly supportive and would be instrumental in my success, too. I didn't know what else to do. I had joined at least twice before in recent years but was always so angry and resentful that I would lose a little weight and then just quit. I'd feel like I was being punished. I definitely felt sorry for myself, and my head was completely in the wrong place. It wouldn't take much to derail me. I would be doing well until I went to a party or baseball game, and I'd want to enjoy myself. I hadn't figured out yet how to have a good time without sabotaging my efforts. It's always been much easier for me to stay on a program when I'm home, but I have to be able to leave the house and enjoy life.

Soon I'd be arguing with myself about whether I should eat a piece of cake or some nachos. Part of me would say, *Don't do it. You know it'll wreck your progress!* The other would say, *You deserve it. You've been 'good.' Eat the nachos!* I'd argue with myself for a while, getting more and more agitated, and then I'd start to feel sorry for myself. Finally, I'd scold myself, *You should be able to enjoy yourself! If you had any willpower at all, you wouldn't be in this situation.* And that is what would start the self-pity and the anger and the feelings of deprivation.

I would fall off the wagon soon. Every single time. I didn't realize that there were ways to fully enjoy life without completely going off the rails. There were strategies I could use to eat, enjoy, and still stay true to my health goals. I know now that mindset is critical to successfully losing weight, to making long-term changes, and to building a sustainable lifestyle. I wish I had known it earlier because first, maybe I would have successfully lost weight much earlier in my life and second, maybe I would have stopped beating myself up years ago.

Of course, I was worried that it wouldn't work. I was afraid I wouldn't be able to lose weight. After all, I had no thyroid, a very slow metabolism, had just had a radical hysterectomy six months earlier, was fifty-eight years old, and postmenopausal. Possibly, I might not be able to lose any weight at all. The odds were definitely stacked against me. My track record wasn't that great. I hadn't really been all that successful at losing weight and I was never successful in keeping it off. Periodically, I would lose fifty or sixty pounds, but I always gained it back plus more. Like so many others, I mainly lost weight by drastically reducing my caloric intake and doing two-a-day workouts at the gym, but I knew that wasn't sustainable. Plus, I was getting too old to do that. This time had to be different.

Chapter Thirteen

I knew I needed help. I had to find a program or some kind of framework to succeed. If I could do it on my own, I would have done it already. I wanted an evidence-based program that I could work into my life. I'd tried other programs that required special food, or that were highly restrictive, and they weren't sustainable for me. I needed to make small, manageable adjustments, not huge, sweeping changes. Those are too hard to keep going. I'd tried it so many times, and it never worked.

I'm not recommending any one program over another. Weight Watchers happened to fit the kind of lifestyle changes I wanted to and felt like I could make, so that's what I did. I had to find something I could do for the rest of my life. I needed something with structure and accountability.

I thought I did a pretty good job of not letting my weight stop me from participating in normal activities. In retrospect, that wasn't quite true. I realized much later in life that I self-censored. I opted out of activities that I thought might be embarrassing, and although I did some things that took guts, like trying out for the pom-pom squad in ninth grade, I didn't attempt activities where I knew I would fail. I don't suppose most teenagers would put themselves in that position; the problem was there were so many things I just couldn't physically do, so I limited myself.

I did make the squad as an alternate, though I wasn't very good. Plus, instead of getting to wear a cute outfit like all the other teams, we all had to have our uniforms handmade because they didn't come in my size. As you can imagine, my fellow team members weren't thrilled.

I've learned over time that I do better with structure and boundaries in my life. Left up to my own devices, I tend to be highly reactive and make emotional decisions instead of rational, logical decisions. This is especially true around food. Admittedly, I'm an addict, a food addict and I'm addicted to sugar. Plus, I'm an emotional eater. That's what I do, not everyone does, but I do. It makes sense now, looking back, that I do better with structure. I didn't have much of it growing up. There was a lot of chaos and very little predictability. In a situation like school, where there was tons of structure, I thrived. In college, it became up to me to create the structure, which I didn't know how to do at that time, so the struggle came back. Without structure, I get overwhelmed and don't know what to do.

So, Weight Watchers it was. I really wanted it to work, because the next step would be surgery, and I absolutely didn't want to do that. I'd tried eating specially created foods produced by weight loss programs, but I couldn't stand the taste. Plus, I knew I couldn't eat just a few freeze-dried meals. Talk about feeling deprived! I also couldn't stand drinking protein drinks. They tasted terrible to me, too, so those were out. I bought books that touted the latest programs, *The South Beach Diet*, *Body for Life*, *The Blood Type Diet* (yep, there was one based on blood type). You name it, I bought the book and gave it a try. It just never worked out long-term. I knew people had found a lot of success with Weight Watch-ers. Plus, you ate normal food, so I wouldn't have to make two sepa-rate meals: one for me and one for Ronn. Ronn does a lot of the cooking, and I didn't want him to have to create separate meals for me. That would have made me feel incredibly self-conscious, and that wouldn't have been good, either.

I was fully aware that successfully creating a new lifestyle meant I had to make some changes. It's hard to know where to start, but clearly, what I was doing wasn't working. I've learned that that's ok. We all have to start from wherever we are. There's some irony here in that I taught Behavior Change Theory to staff at the Centers for Disease Control and Prevention (CDC) for a few years. You would think I would have some clues on how to do this, but I didn't. It goes to show you that information isn't enough to create behavior change.

I did my best to set myself up for success. I prepped my food for the week on Saturday or Sunday. I have standard fare in addition to lean proteins like grilled or smoked chicken, turkey, and salmon. I roast sweet potatoes and butternut squash, I sauté some combination of vegetables that usually includes zucchini, yellow squash, mushrooms, onions, and peppers, and I make sure I have salad greens and fixings on hand. That way, I always have lunch ready to go and healthy sides at dinner. I have instant oatmeal and protein bars in my cabinet at work in case I need a snack. I learned right away that if I don't have healthy options at hand, I make poor choices. Making sure I always have options that support my lifestyle makes decision-making easier.

I don't like kale. I've tried kale every which way, but I just don't like it.

I decided early on that I wouldn't eat food I didn't like just because it was low in calories. I do, however, like hard-boiled eggs, sugar-free pickles, and multigrain crackers but not as a steady diet. I like all those things but if I had to eat only that for the rest of my life just to maintain my weight, I couldn't do it. I'd be miserable. I started buying fresh ingredients and learned how to prepare them in a healthier way. I ate what I loved either by lightening it up or eating a smaller portion. Then, something odd happened; once I started eating more healthfully, my taste buds changed. I had no idea that would happen until one day I roasted some vegetables with some black cherry balsamic vinegar and about lost my mind when I tasted them. My mouth was dancing with joy; my taste buds were in heaven. They were alive!

Who knew it was possible to love roasted vegetables so much?

I realized that I had probably desensitized my taste buds with all the fast food and processed foods I had been eating. It's no wonder I never felt full or satisfied given what I was feeding my body. I never gave my body any nutrients it could use as fuel, so it constantly craved something it could use. My poor body.

I also realized from decades of trying to lose weight, that I was missing an important component. My head wasn't in it. Most challenges are mental, even if the goal is physical. Want to climb a mountain? You need to develop mental toughness to get through the hard days. Want to run a marathon? You have to figure out how to lace up your shoes and train, even when you don't want to or it's raining or cold or you don't feel well. Want to lose weight? The same thing applies.

Without a healthy mindset, I was prone to self-sabotage and could easily talk myself out of doing the consistent behaviors necessary to be successful. I was told once, if you're only 99% in, you'll fail. That 1% gives you an out every time. I had to be in one hundred percent. No excuses. I was tired of being angry at the world for having to lose weight. I was tired of fighting my way through every day to eat healthy. I was tired of being frustrated because my success was always so short-lived. I was just plain tired. There had to be a better way.

Once I began my weight loss journey, I started to see how important the mental piece really was. A big part of it is how I talked to myself. Those tapes in our heads are powerful. Whatever story we tell ourselves, that's our reality. If we keep telling ourselves that we're ugly, disgusting, or don't deserve to have a better life (whatever that means to you), then we can't possibly begin to heal, let alone achieve our goals. If I told myself I couldn't do this, then I couldn't.

How can anyone, who constantly tears themselves down, find the fortitude to keep going? Insulting and berating yourself isn't motivating, it's destructive. Have you ever insulted yourself to success? I haven't.

I believe the reason I made it through PhD school was because I kept slowly building myself up. Believe me, most of us were convinced at some point or another that we weren't going to get through the program. I had to become my own best cheerleader! I couldn't rely on others to constantly build me up. I had to convince myself that I could do it. And once I had a few small wins under my belt, it became easier and easier to see myself succeeding. These triumphs helped me to not throw in the towel when I hit a wall. Past successes helped me rewrite the scripts that allowed me to recognize that I'd done hard things before, and thus, I could do hard things again. Plus, I was constantly building my toolbox by acquiring new techniques and strategies that helped me study, read academic research more efficiently, or improve my writing. None of us have all the tools we need at the beginning to complete a difficult task (if we did, it wouldn't be difficult). It's in the doing that we start learning what we need to succeed. It would have been fantastic if walking through the door at the University of Kentucky, I had possessed all the knowledge, skill, and habits necessary to earn my PhD. That's just not how it works, at least not for me. Most of the time, I had to build the car as I was driving down the road. It's scary, but if I waited until I felt I had everything I needed to be successful, I'd never start anything.

I realized I had to take it one class at a time, sometimes one week at a time, and not look at it from the big-picture perspective. Just as needing to lose over one hundred pounds was overwhelming to me, so was earning my doctorate. There was no way to get through it except by writing one paper at a time, taking each test as it came, and just putting one foot in front of the other. By the time I finally looked up, the semester would be over, and I had another one in the books. All the small wins added up to momentum and progress. I had to address each step, one at a time. First coursework, then qualifying exams, then writing a prospectus, then writing a dissertation, and then my defense. The same would have to be true here. I would have to start with small wins to start building my confidence. If it worked for getting a PhD, it could work with weight loss and building a healthy lifestyle.

To be honest, my issue wasn't so much that I felt I was ugly or stupid. I knew even though I was obese, I wasn't disgusting or gross or unintelligent. However, I did sometimes question whether I was capable of succeeding or whether I deserved a better life. Admittedly, I sometimes called myself stupid or immediately thought I was an idiot because I kept failing at what I considered very basic skills that I felt I should know how to do by this point. It's a bad habit that I'm still working on as I catch myself doing that to this day periodically. For example, I struggle with technology. It doesn't always make sense to me, especially at first, and if I get tripped up, which I almost always do, I immediately become frustrated. If I stopped there, it would be understandable. But no, I end up taking it a step further, berating myself for not understanding technology better, for not knowing more about it than I do.

Make sense? No? It doesn't to me, either.

It doesn't help me in managing those situations, and it certainly doesn't encourage me to enhance my skills. I basically explode, call myself names, and then shut down until Ronn solves the problem. Then, I make sure I tell myself how ridiculous I'm being and become embarrassed. I'm not sure where that particular strategy for dealing with challenges came from, but it's not very productive. I'm working on it, though. It makes me crazy.

I finally realized it's also what we *don't* say to ourselves. I had to get better at telling myself, *Good job, Gretchen. You rocked that! Or, Girl, you gave it everything you had. Take the lesson you got out of it, regroup, and get back in there!* What a difference that would have made early on versus constantly tearing myself down. There are usually some positives in almost any situation even if you don't fully succeed. I just had to learn how not to see everything as black and white.

When I first started Weight Watchers, I had to give myself credit even if I didn't have a perfect eating day. Intellectually, I knew I would have missteps, bad eating days, but I still put pressure on myself to stay as close to the program as possible. What I didn't realize was happening though, was that I was putting so much pressure on myself to never exceed my points (the program uses a point system with a daily allowance along with weekly points that you can use as you wish), that I was becoming increasingly anxious that I might have to at some point. I wasn't sure how to handle that and it turned into real fear.

Weight Watchers has a private platform, similar to Facebook, where members share their thoughts, challenges, successes, questions, or inspiration. I would read where people would eat cheesecake or pizza or something extremely high in points, and they would talk about how much they enjoyed it. They would be celebrating a birthday or an anniversary, and they were enjoying it all, including those high-point foods. I thought to myself, *I could never do that. I would be too afraid I would never stop eating!* Then I thought, *Do you really think you will go the rest of your life never eating a piece of cheesecake or pizza? Do you even want a life where eating a piece of pie or cake fills you with so much anxiety or dread that you couldn't enjoy it if you did eat it?*

My answer was a resounding, *NO!* I realized there will absolutely be times when I will want to choose to enjoy these foods. There will also be times when I might not have a lot of options and have to do the best I could. Either way, I had to figure out a way to not be so anxious about it. Mindful, yes. Anxious or fearful? No.

I still had a lot of work to do. At least I was finally realizing that it would have as much, if not more, to do with my mindset as it did with my physical transformation. In fact, I was figuring out that my weight was directly related to my internal thoughts and beliefs, along with my relationship with myself which was driving everything. Until I did the inside work, the outside was never going to come to fruition. That was a powerful realization. The inside drove my outside.

Chapter Fourteen

About three months into Weight Watchers, Eric called me. It was a Saturday night. I will never forget that call. He told me he had Covid. He had been fully vaccinated, but we both knew he was highly immunocompromised because of the dialysis, his diabetes, and his overall poor health. It was the call I never wanted to get, and he never wanted to make. He was still in assisted living and had finally received his prosthetic leg after a year, but he was too weak to use it. His other foot now had an ulcer that wasn't healing. Deep down, I knew that he wasn't going to get better, he was never going to thrive enough to come down to be with us. We both desperately wanted to be together, but I could never figure out the logistics of getting him from Michigan to Mississippi with all of his health issues. He had to do dialysis every other day or so. How would we do that on the road? Without him being strong enough to walk on his prosthetic, how would I get him in and out of the car or in the bathroom? Moving was all he ever talked about when he was in the hospital. When I would fly home to be with him, I'd walk into the room and the nurses would say, "You're Eric's sister. All he talks about is you and coming to live with you."

The last time I saw Eric, he was in the hospital. He was really sick, and I knew I had to be with him. Even though he was well over six foot tall and looked like a big, tough guy, he was my baby brother, and he needed me there. I did my usual talking to the doctors and nurses but mainly I just sat with him. We talked. He slept. I just held his hand. He always visibly relaxed when I walked into the room the same way I would when he came to be with me when I needed him. We just knew everything was going to be okay if we were together. No matter what.

During this particular hospital stay, he was shuffled between the ICU and the floor, his amazing nurse manager, Rob, made sure Eric and I knew exactly what was going on at all times. Rob did everything he could to make sure Eric was in his unit so he could manage his care. He had a long history with Eric and understood his medical challenges. I always slept better when I knew he was in Rob's care.

Once Eric was on the mend, I told him I had to go back to work. He never liked to see me go, but he never asked me to stay longer. This time he did. He was scared. I extended my visit for a few days, and we just hung out at the hospital, talking and laughing, and I continued holding his hand when he slept. Finally, I had to leave. I didn't want to go, but I had to get back to work.

"Alright, Bud, I gotta go," I said and kissed him on his forehead. I said I loved him, he said he loved me, too. I left. I cried all the way to the airport.

I was devastated when I got the call that he had Covid. I knew what that meant. Surviving it would take a miracle. I had just lost my aunt to Covid. I also worked in a hospital; I knew how serious it was. I told Ronn how worried I was and continued to pray. About a month earlier, Eric had been in the hospital, but this time I didn't have to go home. He wasn't that concerned, but I knew his overall health was deteriorating. Ronn had gone up to Michigan a few months earlier to get the condo packed up, so Eric at least felt that we were working towards getting him down to Mississippi. We thought it might make Eric feel more hopeful. Maybe I needed that more than Eric did. Guilt was eating me up. Ronn saw Eric as he was getting off the transport bus from dialysis. He said he didn't look good, though I chalked that up to dialysis. It is so hard on your body. He had a chance to talk with him later, though, and I was glad he at least got to talk with him.

A month or so before he got Covid, I realized I had to start letting him go. I had to turn him over to God. I was fighting so hard not to lose him, but I knew that wasn't my call. If love was enough to keep him alive, he would live to be one hundred. But it wasn't, and it was tearing me apart. A week or two before he got Covid, I had a long conversation with God.

"I know Eric is sick and he doesn't have much time left. I know I have to turn him over to you so I am. I'm turning him over and know that you'll take good care of him. I know that Mom, Dad, and Chris will be there to welcome him Home, and he won't have any more pain. I have to trust you, Lord."

I cried as I prayed. I knew Eric would be full of joy to be pain-free and to be with Mom, Dad, and Chris once again. But I would be alone and devastated. I was going to have to be okay with that. I wasn't.

When Eric had called that Saturday, he said something totally out of the blue. He said he had made peace with Dad. He'd been thinking a lot and talking to him. I was happy to hear that, and he didn't say much more than that about it. It was a powerful statement, though. Eric and Dad had had a tumultuous relationship their entire lives and Dad had hurt Eric deeply so many times. When he said that, I thought, *He's ready to go.*

In Michigan, there were some crazy laws and requirements put in place around Covid. If you were in assisted living or a rehab facility and contracted the disease, there were only a few places you could go if you didn't require hospitalization. Why they felt he didn't need hospitalization with all of his comorbidities, I will never know, but they transported him to a facility near Detroit. Any time one of my family members was taken anywhere, I was always in constant contact with the hospital or facility. Always. I spoke with someone at the facility where they were taking him, and they admitted that communication was poor there and that I needed to be patient because it often took a while to get to talk to someone.

I said, "Are you kidding me? I'm not going to be ok with that!"

Eric called me on Wednesday, a few days after he arrived in Detroit. He sounded funny. He wasn't quite making sense, and he was getting agitated with me. He was asking me to call them and do something (I don't remember what), but I said I would absolutely take care of it and would talk to him in the morning. I promised him I was on it. He said okay.

"I love you, bud."

"Love you, too, Gretch."

The next morning, I tried to call the facility. I tried time and time and time again. I must have made ten calls that morning, but no one would call me back. I had spoken to the nursing director on Wednesday afternoon who assured me he was doing fine, but she would go in and make sure and call me back. I couldn't get her or anyone else to call me back. I was starting to panic because I couldn't get through to anyone. I called and called and called. Nothing. I was losing my mind with worry.

I was leaving work when I finally got a call from Detroit. *Thank God!* I thought.

"This is Eric's nurse, I'm sorry to tell you that he passed about an hour ago. We did everything we could."

Eric was dead.

"No!! No! No! Not Eric!" I screamed.

As it happened, two of my staff were walking about twenty feet behind me. They both ran to me. Without saying a word, they just grabbed me and held me tight. They wouldn't let me go until they were sure I was okay to drive home. They literally held me up until I got my footing. I was a wreck. I was shaking, but I had to get home. I tried to call Ronn, but he wasn't answering his phone.

I had to call Dave, our funeral director. Dave had handled almost every death in my family. He knew my family well, and I trusted him to handle everything. He told me that Michigan law required him to bury anyone with Covid as quickly as possible. No funerals were being held, of course, but I told him I had to be there when they buried him. Eric wasn't going to be put in the ground without me there. Dave wasn't sure he could put it off that long but would do what he could. He thought he could put it off until noon the next day.

"Dave," I said firmly, "you are not going to bury him without me there. We're leaving tonight and we'll be there in the morning."

He said he'd check in with me in the morning.

I told Ronn when I got home. He was upset, too. I told him what Dave had told me and that we had to get home.

"Ok," he said, "Let's get going."

We were packed and out the door in about thirty minutes. To get there in time, it meant 18-20 hours of straight driving. We left Gulfport, Mississippi at 6 p.m. and Ronn drove through the night. He knew I was in no shape to drive. He drove the entire way. I was free to start processing the loss of Eric. During this time, there had been some kind of gas pipeline issue that was causing a fuel shortage, and the first few stations we stopped at were out of gas. I was panicking. I thought maybe we wouldn't be able to get there after all. I was a mess. I prayed that there would be enough gas stations with gas along the way to get us there. The third station had gas, and we never had trouble finding fuel again.

Dave called me around ten the next morning. He asked how I was doing and where we were. I told him we were less than ninety minutes out and that we would be at the cemetery by noon. Ronn had done it, he had gotten us there in time. He'd been up for well over twenty-four hours, but he just kept driving. Dave said it had taken him longer to get Eric's body than he anticipated so we arranged to meet at the cemetery at three. That would give us time to let people know and even buy some flowers.

When we got to the cemetery, lots of family and friends were there. I had only called a few people and posted what I could on Facebook, but word got around and everyone who could be there was there. They all showed up. That's what we do. Eric was so loved, and everyone was there to support me and say goodbye to him.

A memory had popped into my head during the drive home. I remembered when Eric had decided to move to Miami to be with his girlfriend. He was so young, but he felt it was the right thing to do. I happened to be home, and we were all so sad. Mom, especially. She wasn't going to stop him, though, and neither was I. We all had lives to live, and sometimes that meant leaving Midland. At one point I heard some quiet music playing, it was coming from our music room. I peeked in the room and there was Eric, playing the drums to a melancholy song. He had tears in his eyes, but he was ready to go. It was his turn to spread his wings. Given his relationship with Dad had always been fraught with conflict, he needed to move out anyway. He might as well go where he and his girlfriend could start a new life. I just stood there, with tears streaming down my face. I quietly stepped away. I wiped away my tears and hugged him goodbye. He was ready. But me? Not so much. I wasn't ready to say goodbye on this day, either.

Ronn had to help get me out of the car at the cemetery. I was physically having trouble walking. I just couldn't walk toward the hearse and the grave site. Ronn held on tight, and we walked to his casket. Because of his strength, the friends and family who showed up, and those who held me in their prayers, I had the strength to say goodbye to my best buddy, my heart, my brother.

Chapter Fifteen

I thought for sure losing Eric would derail me, that I would start eating uncontrollably. When he died, I was only three months into my weight loss journey which was hardly long enough for my habits to solidify and become permanent. While I was in Midland, I thought, *I have all the reasons in the world to eat whatever I want. Absolutely no one would think anything of it.* It was tradition to eat at a local pizza place whenever I went home. It was one of the things I looked forward to most when I was in Midland.

But I couldn't. I realized that eating a pizza wasn't going to bring him back, so why bother? I didn't feel like eating anyway. I was too upset. In fact, Ronn kept trying to get me to eat because I just didn't have an appetite. That was unusual considering my go-to coping behavior was always eating. Maybe something was changing, after all. Even though Eric didn't die of complications from his diabetes, his health had deteriorated significantly because of the disease, and it still scared me to death. It continued to motivate me to stay on my program. I didn't eat the pizza, and I was more committed than ever.

I continued to weigh and measure my portions and tracked

what I ate religiously. I had read that tracking was one of the most significant factors in weight loss success, but I also had to be honest. Otherwise, what was the point? So, I tracked everything. Every taste, lick, and bite. At first, I was shocked at how much that added up throughout the day, how much mindless snacking was going on. It started to become clear to me how much I was really eating versus how much I thought I was eating. There was a huge gap there!

I did what a lot of folks do the first week or two on Weight Watchers, I looked up what I had been eating and started adding up the points. Holy smokes! Could I even be that honest about what I had been eating? I wasn't sure I could. It was a lot of food, much of it fast food. When you look up some of those meals, and they can easily come to 45-50 points for one meal, it starts to make sense why I weighed what I did. At that time, the program had calculated thirty points a day for me in order to steadily lose weight. I was eating almost twice that in one meal! That was quite a rude awakening for me. Surprisingly, I didn't judge myself or beat myself up about it, but it did serve as an important piece of information. If only I would have treated other information for what it was: data. That's what my weight was: data. That's what my diet was: data. It was objective information that I could use, not a reflection of my character. I learned this a lot later than I could have. I know I would have saved myself a lot of heartache and blame had I approached it this way before now.

When I finally stopped and objectively looked at what I ate, how much I ate, and when I ate, things started to make more sense. I ate a wide variety of foods, but my portions were huge. Plus, I ate all the time. That was partly due to not ever feeling full. My brain just never communicated to my stomach that I should stop eating, no matter how much I ate. I ate until I was stuffed and uncomfortable, but my brain never would tell me I was full, even when I had consumed what I knew was a substantial amount of food. I was also an emotional eater and addicted to sugar. Any surprise that I was morbidly obese?

Dr. Dimitriades (affectionately known as Dr. D.), prescribed Trulicity, a once-a-week injectable medication to help get my get my A1c down. Along with a healthy diet and some exercise, it was also shown to help you lose weight. It also helped quiet the food noise. This term has gotten a lot of attention recently and I think that's a great name for it. Obesity is a complicated issue and one of the issues is the constant preoccupation with food, which easily leads to overeating. If I wasn't eating, I was thinking about eating. If I was eating, I was thinking about what I was going to eat next. It was a constant loop in my head. I hated it. The medication also helped me feel full which was great because I hated the feeling of hunger. It made me anxious. It helped bridge the time I needed until my stomach physically started to shrink so I wouldn't be starving. I agreed to use it because I wanted my A1c to go down and if it helped me lose weight, that was a bonus. It helped. I lost about thirty pounds in the first three months and my A1c moved into the normal range. After that, we determined I could stop taking it, so I did. I lost the remaining eighty pounds without any additional medication. After a short time, I was able to stop taking Metformin and blood pressure medication, too. My labs were turning around, and I was regaining my health.

I was thinking about what I wanted my goal weight to be and wanted to run it by Dr. D. We were talking in my office one day and I told him what I was thinking.

He considered. "I think that's reasonable," he said. "However, don't be surprised if you don't reach that goal. As long as your labs are good and you're feeling healthy, I'll be happy. You don't have to reach that low of a weight."

He reassured me that from a health perspective, he was thrilled with how I was progressing. If I stayed on course, I would be in a really good place health-wise and that was what was important.

"Watch me," I said.

He just smiled. I don't know why that particular goal weight was so important to me; it was rather arbitrary, to be honest. I wasn't after a certain size, but I had chosen that weight when I lost weight in my twenties, and I had never quite made it. It was important for me to hit that number. I knew as long as my A1c was normal, the rest of my labs were good, and I had energy and was able to do the things I wanted to do, I would be fine no matter what my weight was, but I wanted to try and hit that number: I wanted to lose 110 pounds.

Having to lose over one hundred pounds was overwhelming. Sometimes losing ten pounds can be overwhelming, and the more you have to lose, the more overwhelming it is. I had to figure out a way to not focus so much on the end goal. If I only focused on the big picture, I knew I would get discouraged and quit. So, I broke it down into ten-pound increments. That way, no matter where I was in my weight loss process, the most I ever had to lose was ten pounds. Some break it down into five-pound goals. Whatever works to avoid being overwhelmed is the way to go. Breaking goals into manageable mini-goals is a proven and successful strategy. The old question, "How do you eat an elephant? One bite at a time" applies here.

It worked like this: If my current weight was 237 pounds, I told myself I only had seven pounds to lose. That's it, not 57 or 67 or 107, just 7. As I continued to lose, that 7 became 5.6 and then 3.2 and then I would hit 230.8 and only need to lose 0.8 pounds. Then, I'd start all over again. I would reset the 10-pound goal and as the pounds came off, the number went down. Most of the time, I didn't even have to lose the entire 10 pounds. If I had 0.8 to lose to reach 230 pounds, and I lost 2.1 pounds, it meant I only had 8.7 pounds until the next decade. It probably sounds complicated, but it wasn't. For me, it kept me focused on the present and it worked. Only needing to lose ten pounds or less didn't cause me the anxiety that having to lose over one hundred pounds did. It took away some of the paralysis.

For most of my life, once I started eating, it was hard for me to stop. I found out later that there were several reasons for that, including a serious sugar addiction, but I hated my preoccupation with food. I hated the anxiety I had around food, and I hated being a slave to food. I realized that my brain treats sugar like a drug. The more I ate, the more I had to eat. I had to keep feeding that sugar addiction.

They say in Alcoholics Anonymous that "One drink is too many and a thousand is not enough." The same is true for food, at least it was for me. The problem is that we have to eat. Not eating isn't an option; it's necessary for sustaining life. Therefore, I had to figure out how to eat in a healthy way and live in a world where food is everywhere. A world where food is often our love language and how we show each other how much we care. This was going to be a tough challenge.

After about two weeks of being on Weight Watchers, once I eliminated processed sugars and carbs from my diet, my cravings stopped. They just disappeared. Then something else occurred. I was eating dinner and, suddenly, I didn't want any more food. I stopped eating. I just stopped. I still had food on my plate. For most of my life, I had always finished what was on my plate. This time, I just put my fork down and sat there. I had never experienced that sensation before. There were times when I would overeat and be uncomfortably stuffed, but it wouldn't last long, and I would eat again. This feeling—the feeling of satisfaction and gentle fullness— had never happened before. It finally dawned on me what was going on: I was full. For the first time in my life, my body and my brain were finally working like they were supposed to! I was feeding it nutrient-rich foods that my body needed to thrive, I was eliminating processed sugar and carbs, and it rewarded me with functioning like a normal body should. This was a life-changing moment for me. I could finally start to trust my body. The lights were slowly coming on.

Not surprisingly, I had a lot of conversations with myself over the years. I would beat myself up for being weak, lazy, and undisciplined. I had no idea what sugar and processed carbs were doing to my body and my brain, so I blamed myself, just like the rest of the world blamed me. I spent a lot of time telling myself how useless I was, that I didn't deserve to be happy, that I was worthless because I had zero willpower. After all, I couldn't even control my eating. A cupcake or a bag of chips was more powerful than I was. The world was right, I had little purpose. What some folks don't realize is that while others' words can be harsh, they are nothing compared to how we talk to ourselves. Come to find out, we were all wrong.

Chapter Sixteen

A big part of why I had been unsuccessful in the past was because I was only focusing on the scale. It's easy to do because, ultimately, that was my goal, but that's not where my focus needed to be. Sometimes, it's not even that hard to lose weight, but I needed to figure out the whys. Why was I self-soothing with food? Why did I need healing? Why was I treating myself like this? These were important questions, and I had to find some of the answers. I needed to work on the inside. If I was able to do the hard internal work, maybe the outside would take care of itself.

I also knew I needed accountability, structure, and consistency. As human beings, we tend to underestimate our negative behaviors (how much we eat, drink, or smoke, for example) and overestimate our positive behaviors (how much we exercise, the number of vegetables we eat, or how much sleep we get). The way I saw it, denial got me into this situation, so only complete honesty was going to get me out of it.

I had to begin addressing the real issues that caused my overeating. I knew, and finally accepted, that if I didn't get to the root of my eating, nothing would change, even if I did manage to lose weight. Overeating is a symptom of something else, and I needed to figure out what that was to start healing. Fear is a powerful motivator; it gets our attention. What we choose to do in response is up to us. I made the decision to start doing the hard work.

I realized in short order that I needed some additional help to work on the inside stuff. We all do. I don't believe any of us are supposed to do all this on our own. There are aspects that only we can do, within ourselves. There are other aspects where we need some one-on-one guidance, whether it's through coaching or a therapist, to help us work through some pretty complicated issues. I think we can look to our larger communities to help us with still other aspects of our journey. The point is, I had to figure out who could help me with which parts because I knew I couldn't do it all alone.

I started working with a transformational coach. I had never heard of a transformational coach before, but we found each other, as often happens when you start opening your eyes to the opportunities and possibilities the universe puts in your path. Once again, this opportunity came into my life at exactly the right time. Any earlier and I wouldn't have been open to it or ready to do the work. As it happened, I saw a comment from an acquaintance on a LinkedIn post from Transformational Coach Marcie Montgomery. Between Marcie's post and my friend's comment, it got my attention. I chimed in saying I had never heard of a transformational coach and asked what it was. Marcie responded and offered to meet for a brief virtual conversation. I thought, why not? We connected and I liked her immediately. I felt strongly that she would be able to help me work on some things that needed clarity. She also had a background in working with grief, and I knew I was still working through Eric's death (and Mom and Dad's, for that matter). I thought the combination might be helpful.

Transformational coaching, as I would find out, is about doing a deep dive into the essence of who we are. Not what the world *tells* us we are, not even what we tell ourselves, but who we are in our most pure form. For me, it's become about alignment with the values I hold most dear and walking my true path. It sounds cliché to say, but I've always been searching for my purpose. Not everyone hears this call or is even interested in pursuing such things, but I always have. I've always been a searcher and a wanderer, and it was all starting to make sense now.

I used to wish I had followed a similar path as my friends and peers did. They always seemed to know what they were supposed to do and in what order. I was always jealous of anyone who followed the expected path: graduate high school, go to college, graduate from college, get a well-paying job and make a good living, buy a house, get married, and have enough financial security to retire. I could never seem to find my footing on that path. I was always taking detours and trying something new. My poor mom. I know she dreaded my, "Hey, Mom, guess what I'm going to do?" phone calls that she received on a regular basis.

One of these calls happened when I was in my mid-twenties. I was working in Utah at a ski resort in the winter and a white-water rafting company in the summer. During the off-season, my friends were doing bike tours around the country. I called her to tell her I would be bike-touring through the Colorado Rockies by myself on a mountain bike. Of course, I had to do that. It didn't matter that I had never ridden a bike more than five miles and was in terrible physical shape. I can only imagine what she was thinking when I told her I would be stopping along the way, staying at campgrounds or wherever I found a spot. One night, I saw a Catholic Church open. I stopped and knocked on the rectory door. I asked the priest if I could camp in the backyard. He said sure and kept the church open in case I needed to use the bathroom.

I probably had a couple hundred dollars to do this adventure. The plan was to start from Utah and bike through the State of Colorado. It never occurred to me that I couldn't do this. My friends were doing it, so I thought I could, too. This was before cell phones, so my poor family had to wait until I came across a pay phone to check in. I made it about 300 miles before I ran out of money and energy. I grabbed a bus home with my bike in tow. I had a lot of those adventures during my lifetime. I now know that all the constant adventure-seeking was more about searching for answers externally, rather than looking internally to heal early childhood traumas, embracing self-acceptance, and learning to love myself. I was never going to find what I was looking for in a new town. I needed to look inward.

I didn't know what to expect with my first session with Marcie, but as usual, I jumped in with both feet and heart wide open. I've realized I don't know how else to be. I jump in, I get hurt, I get knocked down and then I get back up to try again. It has never occurred to me to quit. I change course constantly, but I never quit trying to figure things out. Trust me, there were many times I was not on the right path. In fact, frequently, I was absolutely *not* on the right path, but I would soon right myself and carry on. I came to realize through therapy and working with Marcie, that since day one, even as a little girl, I wasn't weak at all, I was strong. And I was resilient.

I also tend to dismiss or diminish my life experiences. I never think about my life as being anything particularly remarkable. It just was what it was or is what it is. I understood that my childhood was challenging, but I wasn't alone. Many people grow up in alcoholic homes or homes with other types of addiction. When I first started working with Marcie, I had to fill out an intake form that covered a lot of material, including, of course, childhood memories and experiences. In there, I wrote about Dad's alcoholism, Chris's hemophilia, Eric's accident, and then later, my having cancer three times, being diagnosed diabetic, and then my physical transformation. Once I put it on paper, I realized it was a lot. Maybe I did have more to process than I thought. Possibly, I was so engrossed in getting through my life that I never took the time to think about everything I went through.

We started where you usually start, at the beginning. I talked about growing up, and what kept coming out of it was how strong, how resilient, I was. I had never thought about it that way, but my therapist, who I started seeing a few months later, would end up commenting on that, too. We spent some time exploring those experiences and talking about how I saw myself now compared to me as a little girl. I finally started to see how strong I was to not only survive some of my experiences, but to not be jaded or bitter because of them. I saw how I kept showing up and putting one foot in front of the other even when, especially when, I had no idea what I was doing or how to do it. And, I did it through significant dysfunction growing up.

I kept going through the bad relationships, too much drinking in my twenties, and an unhealthy marriage in my thirties. I kept going when I got sick, when Chris died, when Mom, Dad, and Eric died. I didn't know how else to be or what else to do. I still don't. I just keep showing up and figuring it out along the way. The difference now is that I have wonderful people helping me find my way.

I realized there were all sorts of other paths I could have taken. I could have used drugs, I could have withdrawn from life. I could have become an alcoholic like my dad and grandpa. I could have self-harmed, or I could have decided I didn't want to even be alive. While I understand that overeating and being morbidly obese is a form of self-harm, I didn't do many of the other things I could have done. I could also have lived a safe life, never taking chances, but I didn't. I could have quit, but I didn't. I regrouped a lot, but I never quit. Ultimately, I found my voice. I found my path. I found the love of my life. I found my purpose and it was all worth fighting for.

The interesting thing is that both of these amazing women—Marcie and my therapist—have never spoken to each other, yet my conversations with them were often parallel but from different perspectives. They both helped me heal my past, find my path, and shine a bright light on my future. As I've said before, I am a big believer that God puts angels in your path when you need them. Sometimes those angels are in human form, sometimes not. Either way, I know I am not walking my path alone, and I know I am blessed beyond measure every day. Even with the ups and downs and detours, I have no idea why I have been so blessed. To say I'm grateful doesn't even begin to cover it.

One of the areas Marcie and I worked on was identifying my values. I wasn't sure why that's what we needed to do first, but I trusted her and the process. I had never thought about what my values were. We started exploring what was important to me and why. It took a while, but we finally identified my values. For me, I valued family, helping others, being seen, and being heard. None of these things surprised me exactly, it did, however, explain why I felt so frustrated most of the time. I asked her once, how would someone who isn't working with a coach or a therapist identify their values. She said by looking for the things that make them the angriest. Those are the times when your values have been stepped on or dismissed. That made sense. The times I found myself the most frustrated or when I seemed to have a short fuse were the times when I was feeling unseen or not heard.

I found this to be the case often in my professional life. As a PhD, it irritated me when others were addressed as doctor, and I was addressed as Gretchen. It typically happened when the other PhDs were men. The first time it happened, I had just graduated PhD school and had my first professional job as a researcher. I was part of a grant application and there listed in the description of the team were several male PhDs, listed as Dr. and then me, the only female, listed as Ms. My experience, my training, and my degree were being ignored and dismissed. It would happen many times at different organizations. I spoke up every time, and they always fixed it. But it was exhausting. Now, I try to preempt it, but it still happens.

Other times, as head of my department, I either didn't have a seat at the table or when I did, I had no power. It wouldn't matter what I said, it wasn't going to impact the outcome. I've learned how to navigate these situations more effectively by speaking up with more authority, providing stronger supporting data or documentation, and tweaking my messaging to make sure I am at least heard. I realized I abhor being dismissed or ignored. I hadn't realized this until I started working with Marcie, but it made sense as to why I got so angry and frustrated.

I'm not saying being dismissed was solely because I am a woman, though broader research bears this out. Part of it was because I was obese; research shows that we are treated differently in the workplace, we earn less than our thin counterparts, and our ideas are often dismissed. The other part, and the part I own, was because I was timid and unsure. *Why should anyone listen to me when I was barely listening to myself? Did I even think what I had to say was important? If I didn't, why would they?* Identifying my values has been a game-changer for me. It has given me a lot of important information about how I move through my life. I can make adjustments more quickly and speak up more firmly now and it has improved my quality of life significantly.

This also explained why I struggled growing up and often felt invisible. I was a middle child. I had no life-threatening situation to compete with the attention Mom had to give my dad or my brothers. Intellectually, I understand that Mom had only a finite amount of bandwidth, but it still hurt, and it fostered a sensitivity to not being seen or heard that I still carry with me to this day.

Early on, Marcie asked me what some of my limiting thoughts were in preparation for one of our sessions. One of them has always been, "I'm too old." I told her that I wish I had figured some of this out sooner instead of when I was sixty.

"Could you have done this before now?" she asked me.

The answer was a resounding, "No." This was one of the most freeing moments for me. The shackles of feeling behind, of it being too late, were removed. There was a lightness about me as I realized that everything was happening just as it should be at exactly the right time. My life was changing, and I could feel it.

I've always been, in my mind, somewhat of a late bloomer. At least I thought I was. I certainly was compared to my peers and society's measure of what it means to be successful. Now, I'm not so sure. They say that comparison robs you of your joy. I agree. I spent a lot of my life comparing myself to others and always fell short.

I realize I could not have done any of this twenty, ten, or even five years ago. I wasn't ready. At this point in my life, after surviving cancer three times, after being diagnosed with diabetes, after transforming my life and losing my family, I realize I am exactly where I'm supposed to be. What freedom, knowing that I am right on time. I'm not too old, and it's not too late to find my purpose, to walk my path. I am becoming unapologetically me, who, by the way, is pretty damn awesome.

Chapter Seventeen

The odds were not in my favor when I started my weight loss journey. The data are clear: between 80 and 95% of people who lose substantial amounts of weight gain it back. *Yikes!* Because the odds were so stacked against me to succeed, I knew I had to show up and work my program daily. I had to be consistent over a long period of time, or I was afraid I would easily get derailed. I had experienced success in the past, but if I wasn't careful, I would find myself gaining all the weight back. It's incredibly easy to do. So, over time, I kept adding small consistent habits that reinforced a healthy lifestyle (or at least maximized the probability of maintaining one). I figured out that packing my lunch made a big difference. I usually eat breakfast and dinner at home, but lunch could be challenging. Packing my lunch gave me control over that meal, too. It was a game-changer. I realized it was important to identify ways I could remain in control without having to figure out something at the last minute in situations where my options may be limited.

I knew I had to build a lifestyle that protected my total health, not just my weight, because it's all interconnected. I had to build an infrastructure for long-term success so that no matter what kind of day I was having, what was going on in my life, and whether or not I was "motivated" that day, I would still be able to stay on track. When you depend on motivation for success, it's like waiting for a bus that may or may not show up. You might make it to work. You might be late. You might just sit there all day. Beyond the initial trigger or event that got my attention in the first place, it wasn't really about motivation at all; it was about the process or infrastructure I was able to put in place. It was quite a different way for me to look at weight loss. I also realized I had to commit and recommit to my health goals every day. This was hard to do but being passive wasn't going to serve me; I had to be intentional and I had to stay focused.

We live in a culture that bombards us with food. Everything is tied to food. It makes life challenging to navigate constant advertising, lunch meetings, holidays, special events, and all of the other things we hold dear. I had to figure out how to enjoy life and still take care of myself. I can't skip every special event from here on out just because I want to maintain a healthy weight. People do it all the time. I just had to figure out how I could do it. I learned that I would do better if I wasn't starving when I attended events where there would be food. I always grab something to eat before I go. That takes the edge off so if there are some healthier options that I want to eat, I could. If I wanted to wait until I got back home to eat, I could do that, too. Sometimes, I decided to dive in and eat a little extra. Whatever I decided to do, it was a conscious choice. I also realized the first few bites of an amazing dessert can be sublime, but the effect diminishes rapidly. So, I started to eat slowly, pause between bites, relish the first few bites, and then stop.

Do I always stop at two or three bites? Of course not! Sometimes, if I'm at a restaurant or at a birthday party and the cake or dessert is extraordinary, I'll eat the entire piece or more. Life is short, sometimes you need to eat the cake! I have learned to make these times special, though. Eating cake every day diminishes the joy of eating cake for me, especially if it's not a very good cake. If I'm going to eat cake, or pie, or a donut, it needs to be a truly delicious one. Why bother eating it if it isn't extraordinary? Sometimes, I even put it on a beautiful plate, too.

One challenge for me was distinguishing between actual hunger and emotional eating. I've always suffered from anxiety. Over the years, I've had to take medication to get rid of the dreads and to stop my mind from racing. When Mom died, I had trouble focusing, and my thoughts would go to a negative place constantly. Everything was bad. I didn't like my job or the city where I was living, and life was awful. I'm sure I was depressed, too. I explained what was going on to my doctor, and he prescribed a low-dose anti-anxiety and antidepressant. I took it for a year or so until everything stabilized and then I was able to slowly get off the medication.

My anxiety still comes around now and again. I knew I had to learn to deal with it, or soon I'd be eating as a coping mechanism again. It was then that I finally realized I needed to work on my relationship with food. I figured if I did that, the scale would follow. It did.

So, I started to work on my relationship with food. I mean seriously and intentionally work on my relationship with food. What did that even mean? I'd heard it said many times, but I had no clue where to start. Obviously, I knew my relationship with food was unhealthy, or I wouldn't be morbidly obese. I decided to start paying attention to my body. As I started listening to my body, really listening, and getting to know its cues, I began to notice a few things. First, sometimes I truly am hungry. I know this because my stomach growls. This was a new sensation to me. Rarely did I ever let myself get hungry enough for my stomach to growl. I was always eating. I hated the feeling of being hungry, it made me anxious. So, now if I'm actually hungry, I eat. That's how it's supposed to work. I can tell when it's true hunger if some lean protein or a piece of fruit is appealing to me. If it's not, I'm not hungry, I'm bored. If I'm hitting the pantry or the refrigerator because I've gotten into the habit of having a nighttime snack, I have a decision to make. If I'm on the verge of being hungry and don't want to wake up in the middle of the night, I'll eat the snack, because if I'm hungry, it will wake me up out of a dead sleep and then I can't go back to sleep. Sometimes I eat that snack, sometimes I don't, but at least I am actively making the choice.

I started to pay attention to what I ate, when I ate, and why I was eating. I was trying to nail down what triggered my overeating so I could find the patterns. Was it when I was tired? Was it when I was sad or when I had to have an uncomfortable conversation? What needed to be healed? The reasons why I treated my body with such disrespect are complicated. Joining Weight Watchers helped me become aware of what I put in my mouth because I had to track what I ate. Like so many of us, I had no idea I was eating that much. In fact, if you asked me to recall what I had eaten at the end of a day, I would have missed a significant number of calories. It is easy for me to mindlessly eat and not realize how often I did it or how much I ate. I had been mindlessly eating and self-soothing with food for almost sixty years; it was going to take a while to get a handle on it. I was okay with that. I didn't put a time restriction on my weight loss. I didn't put the pressure on myself to lose one hundred pounds in a year or even two. I figured it would happen however it was going to, my emphasis had to be on building a healthy lifestyle and figuring out why I was always turning to food. That was going to take some time.

I still eat all the time, but now, it's in smaller portions and a completely different diet. It's incredibly easy to grab a bag of chips and eat them while watching TV. Before I knew it, the bag was gone. For me, one bag equaled one serving, no matter the size of the bag. So, I knew I would have to track honestly and religiously. I still snack while watching TV (I know, it's still a bad habit). I just plan for it now, and usually (not always), snack on healthier options. One of my strategies to control portions is to count out one serving of whatever I'm eating, and I mean the actual serving size on the label. If the serving size is twenty-four bite-sized chips, that's what I count out and put them in a bowl. If I want more, I have to get up, get the bag out of the pantry, and count out twenty-four more chips. That simple action usually stops me from eating more because it's enough conscious effort to make me think about it. Plus, I have to get up off my couch to do it and sometimes it's just not worth it. You should hear some of the conversations I have with myself. Even I have to laugh sometimes because of how much I talk to myself about food. *Gretchen, do you really want to eat that? Are you truly hungry? You don't even like marshmallows, why are you reaching for them? Put those back. Good grief.*

I still have to tell myself to stop when I'm tempted to mindlessly eat. I sometimes actually have to say, right out loud, "You're not hungry. You're bored. Stop."

While it sounds silly, it works. It's a constant battle, but it got easier as I developed techniques to break the habits that got me to this point. I usually can't just sit there and watch TV anymore. I always have a book or my phone (which is a whole other addiction), typically both. It gives me something to do with my hands and engages my mind, which keeps my mind off food. Other people I know knit or crochet or paint. Frankly, it isn't unusual for me to randomly get up and walk into another room or tidy up my closet or a dresser drawer for five minutes; anything to distract me from thinking about food and eating. Since being on Weight Watchers, the constant preoccupation around food has diminished greatly, but it still shows up from time to time. It's one of the biggest freedoms I have experienced. I use that energy now on more productive endeavors and that was worth the price of admission.

Something I've learned about myself throughout this process is if I get too hungry or too tired, I make poor decisions. I just do. I suppose that's true for a lot of people. I guess that's the definition of hangry. If I get too hungry, there's not enough food out there to fill me up. If I make sure to eat a snack when I'm on the verge of getting hungry, it's easier for me to stay the course. I don't know why, but I've never liked the feeling of being hungry, and I absolutely don't like the feeling of being over-hungry. I become really cranky and extremely anxious. I'm a little more comfortable with it now but I still can get a little panicky, especially if my options are limited. That's why I usually have a low-point snack in my purse or bring a small cooler on the road filled with nutritious options. Whether it's an apple and a piece of low-fat cheese, a protein bar, or beef jerky, I make sure I don't get to the point of getting too hungry. Ronn always double-checks that I have snacks before a trip. I think it's self-preservation for him.

I can only focus on eating one meal, one snack, one day at a time because if I had to worry about next week or next month or (and this will definitely trip you up), thinking about never getting to eat a cheeseburger or pizza again, I would have quit. I realized early on that I had no intention of giving up my favorite foods for the rest of my life. I certainly wasn't giving up enjoying holidays and birthdays and special events. I was just going to have to learn how to incorporate them into my new lifestyle. I tend to avoid some foods, like fast food, because I don't like how it tastes now, but if it was important to me to eat it, I'd fit it in. Today, I still eat pizza and hamburgers and French fries and pie. I just eat less of it, and I don't do it that often. There's a gift in doing that, though. It makes it more special when you do have it.

Once a year, I eat a pumpkin spice donut. It ushers in the beginning of fall for me. Now, I love a donut. Good donuts, bad donuts (is there really such a thing?), all donuts. Always have, but they're full of sugar, and we all know I'm addicted to sugar. It messes up my body and my mind. For now, however, I still like my annual ritual of eating my fall donut. When I decide to eat that donut, I buy a really good pumpkin spice donut. I eat it slowly, and I savor it. I do the same thing at Thanksgiving when I make my two, small mincemeat hand pies. I eat one the night before and one with Thanksgiving dinner. If I want more, I have to get out the pie crust I made, pull out the rolling pin and pastry mat, roll it out, put it together, put everything away, and bake them. It works great because I usually have no desire to do all that. If I do, it means I really want it. That's just fine, but I only make one at a time. Eating mincemeat pie is a celebration for me and it brings with it all of the good feelings of times past with my mom and family Thanksgivings. It brings back the magic of the holidays and I have no intention of giving that up.

I have taken great care in creating my new lifestyle, but it can still be overwhelming to think about doing this forever, even with a positive attitude and trying not to project too far in the future. Old habits die hard and sometimes I miss the old, comfortable habits. Who doesn't like digging into a huge bowl of ice cream when you're upset or devouring an entire plate of nachos to celebrate your sports team winning? That's why I continue to touch base with myself and ask, *Does this support my goals?* or *Is this something I can eat long-term? Is it delicious enough to make the cut?* If not, I keep finding new recipes or I tweak the current one. I want my diet (as in the food I eat, not a restrictive eating plan) to be more delicious than anything I was eating before. That way, I'll always look forward to my next meal and that's exactly what has happened.

AA and Al-Anon use a book called, "One Day at a Time." I have used that book my entire life. It came in handy during this journey, too. Sometimes, focusing too much on the future gets to be overwhelming, so I would keep breaking things down into increments I could handle. If focusing on my week was too much, I focused on one day. If the entire day was too much, I focused on one meal or one snack. There are a lot of moving parts when you're building a healthy lifestyle, and I couldn't focus on all of them at the same time. So, I kept breaking it down until it wasn't overwhelming to me. Given that I was building my lifestyle, I had to do what worked for me. It didn't matter what other people were doing. I had to find the pieces to my own puzzle and start building.

When I first started my weight loss program, I only focused on what I was eating. I knew that exercise and movement were important, of course, but I also knew that getting control of my eating was going to be key. You can't outrun the fork. I've noticed over the years that there are two groups of people: the ones who get a handle on the food part but struggle with exercise and those who can work out for hours but struggle with the food piece. I am the former. The few times I tried to incorporate formal exercise into my day, it tripped me up. I got frustrated and overwhelmed because the only way I thought I could do it was to wake up at 4:30 a.m. and go to the gym before work. While I could see positive changes and it felt good, it became too much for me. I learned over time that I was increasing my movement naturally throughout my day and that was going to have to be good enough until I could figure out how to build more strength training into my life in such a way that didn't consume all of my free time. We live out in the country now, and I'm finding all sorts of ways to build strength and incorporate more movement into my day and that's good enough for me, for now.

When I look back at my weight loss trends, I rarely lost a large amount after the first few months. While it was exciting to lose four or five pounds in a week, that wasn't going to happen all the time. In fact, I would lose a few pounds at most, then stay the same for a few weeks, or even have a small gain. Even though I never strayed from the program and stayed 100% on point, I didn't always lose. It was disappointing at first, but over time, I realized that my body was going to lose at the rate it was going to lose. The more you lose, the harder it is for you to continue to lose. Sometimes your body just doesn't want to let the weight go.

I came to peace with the weeks when I didn't lose. It helped that I wasn't weighing in somewhere, it was in my own home. I find it incredibly stressful to jump on a scale in front of someone who then records it. I don't like doing it at the doctor's office, either. I realized that our bodies pretty much do what they want when they want. It really is a complex process when you are losing weight and sometimes our bodies fight it. Sometimes, it wants to hold on tight. During my weight loss, I often heard people from Weight Watchers ask what they were doing wrong, frustrated at staying the same for a week or two. My answer was always, "Probably nothing." Our bodies do what they do. I figured if I kept working on my relationship with food, showing up every day, and tracking my meals and snacks, the scale would eventually follow. It did.

Everyone's journey is their own. Everyone has their own weight loss approach, and our bodies respond uniquely. What I did might not work for someone else. Was it hard to see other success stories where they lost more weight faster? Sure, but, in the end, as long as I was showing up every day, I knew I would ultimately reach my goal. I never set a timeline, and I never really thought about how long it would take. I had no idea how long it would take and, frankly, it didn't matter to me. I was already experiencing health benefits beyond the weight loss, and I liked how I felt. I was working hard on my relationship with food and building habits that reduced the anxiety around food and that was more important to me than even losing the weight. I found the cleaner I ate, the happier my body (and brain) were.

I'm addicted to sugar, not everyone is. I know people who can eat fast food and still reach their goals. I know folks who drink a lot more alcohol than I do and still maintain a healthy lifestyle. I know others who exercise regularly and then eat way more than I do. The point is that everyone's body is different, and their choices around food are different. Thus, people lose weight at different rates, and sometimes it takes us more than one or two (or ten) attempts before we figure it out. Comparing our journey to someone else's is a recipe for disappointment and frustration. Keeping my eye on my own journey brought a kind of peace and focus that was necessary to fully explore all the facets of what my new life should be and what worked especially well for me.

"It's not a diet, it's a lifestyle." People throw that statement around a lot, but I finally took it to heart. I never wanted to do this again. I had to build a lifestyle that worked for me every day, through the holidays and special events, through the days I felt good and the days I felt bad, through all the ups and downs of life. That's easier said than done. It takes constant intentional thought, hard work, forethought, and a lot of tweaking. A sense of humor doesn't hurt, either, combined with a whole lot of grace and self-kindness.

There's a fine line between being kind to yourself, loving yourself, and allowing yourself to give in to excuses and denial. It's critical to hold ourselves accountable, but we can do it in a way that is both honest and kind. They aren't mutually exclusive. Beating myself up was counterproductive. Denial was counterproductive. Both are destructive and do not support building a healthier life. Justifying the behaviors as to why I did or didn't do something just fed into the dysfunction that got me here. The trick was being completely honest with myself while using supportive language to move through the challenges. If you tend to beat yourself up, try doing the opposite and see if the results change. It's a hard habit to break but it's key to building your new healthy life.

I am overly honest. Sometimes to a fault. I knew sneaking food or not tracking what I ate would hurt only me. My body is still tracking it, and pretending I didn't eat doesn't support my goals. If you're hungry or want something, eat it, but don't pretend it didn't happen. If you're so inclined, and I always am, figure out why you felt the need to eat if you weren't hungry. Again, eating when we're not hungry can be a strong cue that something more is going on. I like to figure it out so I can make healthier choices next time. It's just too easy to turn a small indulgence into deciding to quit. Part of that is the "all or nothing" mentality that many of us have. If I blow it (in my mind) by over-eating, then I might as well eat what I want the rest of the day, weekend, or week. This is dangerous thinking. Not only do we have to deal with the extra weight, but a lot of guilt often follows. If you're going to eat it, eat it without guilt. What's the point of enjoying something if you're going to feel bad about it?

It takes all the joy away. Set up boundaries so you can get back on track with whatever healthy eating plan you subscribe to. Early on, I think I needed to splurge a little to make sure I had developed the tools to get myself back on track. I needed to build my confidence. Without that confidence, I would have become more and more anxious worrying about what would happen if I wasn't able to eat exactly what I planned. That was causing me to become a little obsessive, and I didn't like that feeling, either. There were going to be situations where I didn't have as much control, and I had to learn how to do the best I could and then get back on track as soon as possible. I had to build those skills. I've lost significant amounts of weight numerous times; I know how easily five pounds turn into a hundred-pound gain. It happens remarkably fast.

For the record, even as I followed my weight loss program carefully, I wasn't perfect. I was never striving for perfection, anyway. It's too much pressure. I'm not a perfect person. Even though I have been successful, I've had my missteps, and I have made my share of mistakes. I often got frustrated and disappointed. It wasn't all rainbows and unicorns. It still isn't. Having a mindset that favored gratitude and understanding that time was a gift that not everyone had helped a lot. It grounded me. It got me through the harder times, along with therapy and coaching. It makes sense that navigating this journey with a more positive mindset would be more helpful than going through the hard times with a negative mindset on top of it. It's not a wonder that I didn't succeed in the past because that is exactly how I did it. Also, I tended to do this all alone and that was making it much harder. As I've gotten older, I've realized that having a team around you, a really supportive team that helps make you stronger, makes anything you're doing more doable. It's not a one-way street. I'm a member of other peoples' teams, too. It's what we all should be doing, supporting each other and helping each other live our best lives.

It's a great feeling to be successful at losing weight, of course. Obviously, it's a highly visible journey. At some point, everyone will notice, and some will comment on it. I'm not sure when it became socially acceptable to comment on anyone's weight or whether it's more or less acceptable than it was previously, but it's often the topic of discussion. Especially as women. As challenging as it's been for me, I can't imagine how much more brutal it is for people in the public eye when magazine covers are dedicated to such things. It boggles my mind.

It took about sixteen months to lose 110 pounds, but I did it. I remember the day I hit my goal weight. It was kind of anti-climactic. I'd been working at it for well over a year and the day I lost my last pound or two, I just smiled. I pumped my fist in the air, and I said, "Yes, I did it!" I had a huge smile on my face. I told Ronn and he congratulated me.

To Ronn's credit, he'd never said anything about my weight. He loved me no matter what, but I loved me more. Not because I lost weight, but because along the way I started loving myself more. The process provided me an opportunity to work on myself, to do the inside work that was necessary to deal with what was causing me to treat myself with less respect and love than I deserved. That's the key. Once I started loving myself, my eating fell in line. I didn't have to self-soothe with food anymore. I was healing and that felt way better than how I looked.

I felt amazing and I had so much energy! My skin was lighter and when I looked in the mirror, I looked twenty years younger. I even had to get new headshots taken because my looks changed dramatically. I must admit, the transformation was remarkable. Truth be told, I love those pictures, but the true transformation was taking place inside.

I realized recently that one of the biggest gifts that has come out of my journey, and the work I've done both inside and out, is that I have learned to trust myself. In essence, I quit letting myself down. Now, when I make a promise to myself, when I set a goal, no matter how big or how small, I know I will keep my commitment to myself. I will show up, I will keep trying, I won't quit and when I achieve it, I will acknowledge it. If I fail, and that happens, I will still celebrate and be proud. No more disappointing myself and no more dismissing my accomplishments. I am learning to celebrate every-thing that is me and, most importantly, I have become proud of who I was and who I am. I am learning to honor myself by treating myself with the care and respect I have always deserved from me. It's funny how that translates into how others treat me, as well.

I think some believe that once you reach your goal, the hard part is done. It's not. It's just the beginning of the journey. Mainte-nance can be challenging. I find I have to continuously evaluate what's working and what's not and then tweak whatever needs tweaking. The danger is in becoming complacent, thinking, *I got this.* Years of losing weight and then gaining it all back and then some should have told me something, but I recently learned an important lesson. Probably one of my more important lessons thus far.

Chapter Eighteen

I had joined Weight Watchers at least twice before. I would lose thirty pounds and then on some beautiful, blue-sky day, I would just stop. Then I would gain the weight back and more. Previous attempts at losing weight were unsuccessful for a lot of reasons and mostly, it was in my head. I felt I was being punished. I felt sorry for myself (this was a BIG one), I was angry, and I always treated it as a diet, something negative I had to do. It was restrictive and, frankly, the food wasn't interesting or tasty. I knew I had to do something different this time. Cliché as it is, I realized I needed to build a lifestyle that was sustainable, but mostly, it had to be delicious and allow me to fully participate in life, and that meant holidays, birthdays, vacations, spontaneous road trips, and times when life threw me curves. This meant I couldn't become so inflexible that the only place I could be successful was if I was at home. I had to create my new lifestyle, so it fit everywhere.

This mindset was freeing. Instead of self-pity and beating myself up for gaining weight again, I started approaching each meal as an opportunity to reach my goals. Was what I was eating helping me reach my goals or not? Would it derail me or empower me?

Gratitude permeated every meal and snack. I know it sounds corny, but it was true. I was reframing how I looked at food and what I was eating. After watching my brother's experience with diabetes, I was just damned grateful I had time. I still approach my health with gratitude, and that has kept my attitude much more positive. I never wanted to be that person who was on a diet and miserable so everyone else had to be, too. I had been that person and hated to admit it. Now, I wanted to be able to eat healthy and live with abundance. I wanted to celebrate life, not just survive until I died.

I got into the habit of prepping food for the week. I was incredibly lucky, Ronn was always willing to throw some chicken on the grill or a turkey breast on the smoker to make sure I was set for the week. It was a big adjustment for him, too. As usual, I made the decision to join Weight Watchers based on my needs and didn't say anything for a few days. A decision like that doesn't just affect me, it was going to change how we both ate, and in retrospect, I certainly should have said something that night, but I didn't. I just started buying fresh fruits and vegetables, lean meats, and other healthier options. When I finally said something a few days later, he was, as expected, supportive. It was my pattern to make decisions without saying anything, even when they affect other people, and then announce them out of the blue. While it's my body and I have the right to make decisions to support a healthy lifestyle, I am married to an amazing man who deserves a heads-up when I'm thinking of making significant changes. I should have said something sooner so we could talk about how to move forward together.

Ronn understood why I was so scared when I was diagnosed with diabetes. He was by my side many times when Mom, Dad, or Eric was in the hospital. One time during a visit to Michigan, Mom was in the emergency room, Dad was already admitted to the same hospital and Eric was home sick. He experienced firsthand how stressful it was trying to navigate all of it. I have dealt with serious health issues since childhood and all throughout my adult life. He understood why I had to do something.

I'm not sure why I didn't tell him right away. Maybe because I was in shock and processing being diabetic. Maybe I was embarrassed. Whatever the reason, I love to cook and figured I would just take over some of the cooking responsibilities. I didn't think about all the other ways it could impact our day-to-day lives. I grew up cooking because both Mom and Dad worked, and it helped take some pressure off Mom, which I tried to do. We often had a large garden, so we usually had food even when money was tight. Mom also canned a lot, which sustained us through the cold Michigan winters. Since I usually helped, I learned how to can, too. My dad and brothers hunted, so Mom ended up canning venison, squirrel, rabbit, and even racoon. I remember eating a lot of wild game dinners growing up.

Some of our best conversations were when we were canning, and I was elbow-deep in crushed tomatoes. It was hard work, and it took all day, but I also had Mom to myself, and I loved that. That was sacred time to me. I was so tickled (and so was Mom) when I passed this knowledge on to Branwyn and now, Branwyn and I have a lot of wonderful conversations when we do this, too.

After I had lost all my weight, a television station in Mobile, Alabama approached me. They wanted to do a story about my being a three-time cancer survivor and my physical transformation after being diagnosed with diabetes. They thought my story was inspiring. I had one day's notice, and they would come to me. I was nervous, but I thought telling my story might help both cancer survivors and people who had a lot of weight to lose, so I agreed to do it. The problem was, other than Ronn, we had only told Eric about the cancer, no one else knew. We hadn't told any of our friends or family about it, and now it was going to be broadcast on TV. I had to tell Branwyn.

I wasn't as concerned about my friends. They'd have to understand that it was just something we wanted to keep private. Sometimes you don't want to share everything with everyone. But I regretted that I hadn't told Branwyn the whole truth. She was married with a young son and had a lot on her plate. I talked with Ronn about whether or not to say anything. I wanted to, my instincts said I needed to, but he didn't want to worry her. I understand that. A parent's first instinct is to protect their children, no matter how old they are. Having kept critical information about previous cancer diagnoses from my family before, I knew how hurt and angry she would probably be. You would have thought I would have learned my lesson but, no. As her dad, Ronn knew her best, so I deferred. I should have told her. We told her what we had told everyone else: I was just having a hysterectomy. No big deal.

Branwyn is a compassionate, loving, and sweet young woman. She's smart and beautiful and strong. I know I'm biased, but I love her heart and how giving she is. I know she would have done anything for me. If nothing else, because of distance, she would have checked in on me daily, prayed for me, and probably sent care packages. By not letting her know what was really going on, I denied her that. Also, it made it seem as if we didn't trust her to be able to handle this kind of bad news. I knew she would be worried because she loves me, but she's mature. Heck, she's a mom, too. She would want to know.

I was sick to my stomach, but I had no choice, I had to make that phone call. I'm pretty good at difficult conversations but this one was tough. I kept rehearsing what I wanted to say before I called her. Ultimately, I just told her what I needed to tell her. I told her how awful I felt, and that I would understand if she was angry. She was. She was also hurt but she forgave me. One of the many qualities I admire about Branwyn is that she speaks her mind. She doesn't candy coat anything. Every once in a while, over the years, we've had to have hard conversations, but it's always done from a place of love.

She still brings it up periodically, mostly to make sure there's nothing else lurking in the background. I think. I don't blame her, though. I knew how hurt Mom and Eric were when I kept my Stage IV cancer diagnosis from them. For some reason, it's a hard lesson for me to learn.

As cancer patients, we struggle with a lot of decisions and who we want to share our news with, and which details we want to share are big ones. Ultimately, a cancer journey, any illness journey, is a personal one. Any serious illness means going down a road that can be uncertain, painful, scary, and emotional. It is up to the patient to decide how much they want to share and with whom. There are pros and cons to whatever you decide, though. Not choosing to share my cancer diagnosis with Branwyn was a mistake. By not doing so, I missed an opportunity for us to become even closer. She didn't hold it against me even though she could have. I'm sure some of my close friends were hurt, too.

My weight loss journey might have been easier had I learned this lesson earlier. I would have had even more support had I told people what I was doing. Obviously, those who saw me every day knew I was losing weight, but I didn't tell anyone else. Part of the reason was because if I failed, it wouldn't be such a public failure. How many times had I made bold pronouncements that I was going to do something and failed? Too many to count. This time, I didn't tell anyone, other than Ronn, until I was ready and comfortable that I would succeed. I never said anything to friends and family on social media until I had lost over seventy-five pounds.

While I think you will understand that train of thought if you have ever dieted and regained weight repeatedly, I also missed out on support. Looking back, I stand by my decision (except I should have said something to Ronn sooner) but everyone needs to do what is right for them.

Chapter Nineteen

Speak up. Speak out. Live your life loudly! Your life is as important as everyone else's! I'd been told this a million times; I just didn't believe it. One of the things I had to learn to do was to speak up and put my needs out there. I used to think that people who loved or cared about me should know what I wanted or needed. Not so! To be honest, most of the time I didn't even know what I wanted or needed, how would they? I realized I was being manipulative and maybe even abusive by not speaking up and then being upset when they didn't accommodate my needs. Sometimes I would just shut down and not say anything. That's even worse.

I knew it wasn't a healthy way to interact with people, especially those I cared about, but I didn't know how else to engage when I was hurting. In the past, I wouldn't say anything if I was uncomfortable or needed something. Now, I'm much more vocal. I couldn't blame others for not knowing what was important to me if I didn't say anything. Playing the martyr wasn't a productive behavior, so I had to learn to be assertive to make sure my needs were being met along with everyone else's. This wasn't easy for me to do.

I think that's true for a lot of people; putting our needs first is just uncomfortable. I finally realized that if I didn't, I would continue to struggle with my health goals. My life depended on making sure I stayed healthy. My self-esteem was just going to have to catch up.

About a year after I reached my weight loss goal, I decided to do a podcast. It was born out of a conversation I had with Dr. Rickey Chance, a family physician I worked with. He asked me one day if I was going to do a podcast because if I was, he would prescribe it to his patients. I thought he was kidding, but he wasn't. He told me that he was astounded at not only how quickly I had lost weight but how my attitude stayed so positive and how I've continued to keep it off. He thought others might benefit from my story. That got me thinking. It might be even more helpful to talk with experts about all the other stuff that impacts our health and gets in our way, too. It wouldn't just be about losing weight; I could explore how it all fits together. It's well known that our physical health is not separate from our mental, emotional, or spiritual health, it's all connected. Maybe if I explored these topics, we could all learn together how complex our health is and then focus on the daily habits and actions we could take to reach our goals. We all love a good transformational story, including the "before" and "after" pictures we see in magazines, but I never really understood the work necessary to get from the before to the after. Now, I was going to find out. In sum, I wanted to focus on the work we have to do in between, both the internal and the external. *The Work in Between* was born!

Since then, I've completed the first season and we're already in over twenty countries. It seems to be resonating with folks and I'm grateful for that. Every time I have a conversation with one of my guests, I learn something new or an action that I can take that helps me. That's one requirement I have on my show, guests have to offer two or three actions we can take that will make a difference over time. It's not enough to just talk about stuff, we have to take action. That's the key!

Losing weight isn't easy and maintaining is just as challenging, but in a different way. Research shows that a huge percentage of people who have lost significant amounts of weight regain it within a few years and then some. Being a three-time cancer survivor, diabetic, over sixty, post-menopausal woman means the cards are stacked against me, for sure. I have to be even more diligent to make sure that I protect myself. It's so easy to lose focus, to be fooled into thinking, *I've got this!* This is especially true once you've reached your weight loss goal, when the pressure to continually lose weight is gone. Also gone is the thrill and excitement of seeing that number drop. That's surprisingly addicting. It's replaced by reinforcement that you're doing what you need to do to maintain your weight. It's not the same rush, but I'm proud of my accomplishment. I still get a great feeling when I stay within my range. It never ceases to make me smile. It's usually followed with an emphatic, *"Yes!"* So, I remain diligent.

After losing over one hundred pounds, my self-image changed. It had to. Some people never quite make the transition from being an obese person (or, in my case, a morbidly obese person) to a healthy person. As I started losing weight, I would catch reflections of myself, and I would stop and look. At first, it would take me by surprise. I remember my first Zoom meeting at work after I had reached my goal. I had trouble focusing on the meeting because I was mesmerized by my picture. I looked so different! I was a thin person!

The first time Dr. Pierce saw me at my goal weight, she walked in and said, "You're a thin person!" I sure was.

That, I admit, took a long time to reconcile in my brain. I slowly made the transition, though, and while I no longer see myself as a fat person, I still have my moments. The first time I flew after losing a significant amount of weight, the old familiar worry as to whether the seat belt would fit or if people would look at me hoping that I wasn't the one sitting next to them would kick in. I catch myself now and remember that I'm not that person anymore.

Going through cancer sucks. Being diagnosed with diabetes sucks. Being morbidly obese sucks. While some illnesses and diseases are more serious than others, each has its own personality, and we all have our own journeys through them. One would think I would be grateful every day I wake up and I am, but there's another side to being the only one left standing: Survivor's guilt.

It was during therapy that I finally realized that I carry a lot of survivor's guilt. In retrospect, I suppose it should have been obvious, but it wasn't. I've lost so many family and friends. It occurred to me one day, I've had cancer three times, yet I'm still here. Standing at the graveside seeing your mom, dad, and both brothers' headstones next to each other is crushing. Yet, I'm still here. I'm happy to still be here but I sometimes question why.

I have survivor's guilt because while I have had my own burdens to bear from cancer and diabetes, I don't fit the narrative of a cancer patient or a diabetic, for that matter. In our culture, the narrative tends toward the cancer patient who has lost their hair, is taking chemo and radiation, spends a lot of time in the hospital, and rings the bell when they are cured. I don't have any pictures of myself in the hospital, I never thought to take them. I didn't lose my hair to chemo or radiation. I never rang a bell. I was very sick at times, and I still suffer from the effects of my treatments. Yet I have survivor's guilt.

What I'm saying is that I feel some guilt for not having lived the stereotypical cancer story. When I say I'm a cancer survivor, people automatically assume I had breast cancer. I always have to clarify. Outwardly, I'm not sure anyone would have ever known I had cancer. How could I get cancer three times, including Stage 4, and survive when others, just as worthy, if not more so, don't survive once? I ask myself, *Why? Why* am *I still here when so many have died? Why am I still here after being morbidly obese, having high blood pressure and a host of other health problems, surviving when others, many much younger than me, did not?* Why, indeed.

The same questions exist around diabetes. Don't get me wrong, I'm very proud of myself for making changes earlier rather than later. Because I took action immediately when I was diagnosed with diabetes, I didn't have to take insulin, lose a limb or my eyesight, and I hope I never do, but so many others have experienced terrible outcomes. I'm grateful I never have, but I am sensitive to the fact that I survived when many have not. Of course, it's not lost on me that I was prediabetic for over five years. It is unfortunate that I didn't make changes then, when I could have avoided additional health problems, but I've quit beating myself up over it.

Ultimately, I have survivor's guilt because so many others, who were loved as deeply as I am, if not more, who had so much more life left to live, are not. I have survivor's guilt because so many of the ones I've held so deeply in my heart are gone. I know they are still with me. I feel them. I talk to them. Every day when I wake up, when I open my eyes and take my first deep breath, they are there. They are with me through the good times and the bad times, but I still have survivor's guilt.

In essence, I have survivor's guilt because I did not suffer as much as others have had to suffer. In my mind, anything I went through was minor compared to others because I lived. I'm still working through this. I still ask myself, *Why me?*

I was pretty messed up when Eric died. I knew I would be. I was so angry. I knew it would hit me hard, but even though I had been preparing for the immense sadness I would feel that day, the anger took me by surprise. We both knew he didn't have a lot of time left given all his health problems. I always felt that I could and should have done more, especially for Eric. I should have been able to move him to be closer to us. Even if he didn't have much time left, especially if he didn't have much time left, it was all he wanted. I couldn't make that happen for a host of reasons. That will always haunt me. I still cry about it, especially late at night after we've gone to bed. If I can't sleep, I talk to him, and I always apologize. I know he's forgiven me, but even as I write this, the tears fall. Loving people deeply means missing them even more when they're gone. For now, I'm able to put most of my guilt on the shelf and carry on. Everyone once in a while though, it creeps up on me. At least, I know what it is.

When people find out that I'm a cancer survivor, a three-time cancer survivor at that, they find it remarkable. I understand that. While I freely and openly talk about it, I'd never talked about it to an audience until recently. I never thought there was a story there to tell. But now, I realize that having navigated and survived cancer is one of the most important parts of the story. That's the story I need to tell because it gives people hope. Because talking about advocating for yourself, finding joy or purpose when you're sick, and learning how to control the parts you can control is important. So is talking about how to communicate with physicians and nurses and your family and friends. That's important, too. So, that's why I'm talking about it and writing about it now. It's helped me be at peace with the fact that I'm still here.

Once I launched my podcast "The Work in Between," I started posting about it on LinkedIn for visibility. I wanted to get it out there so I could start building an audience. In my profile, it says I'm a three-time cancer survivor, which was also starting to get some attention. A few months later, I received a message from Robert Pardi. Rob introduced himself and sent a link to a *New York Times* article that had been written about him and his wife. He thought maybe I would be interested in her story because I was a cancer survivor. She had been diagnosed with an aggressive form of breast cancer at a very young age. She was pursuing an MD/PhD when they found it. After she passed, Rob wrote a book, *Chasing Life*, which I highly recommend. Grief can be a brutal path to walk, and I was still walking mine. I didn't realize it, but I was getting angrier and sadder. I was struggling to put on a happy face. Then Rob reached out to me out of the blue. I read the article and then I read his book. I invited him to be on my podcast. As a rule, we don't talk a lot about grief in our culture, at least not as much as we need to, and I knew this would be a topic that would be helpful to me and my audience.

At some point in my research, I read that he had asked himself, *What is the most amazing thing that could come from this?*, referencing his wife's death and the journey that went along with it.

That stopped me cold. In an instant, grief was reframed for me. I was still sad and angry and all those other emotions, but now, I was thinking about losing Eric in a whole different way. It finally came to me. The most amazing thing that could come from this is my telling his story to help others avoid the same experience with diabetes. The most amazing thing that could come from this is that I could help others realize they can make the changes necessary to avoid preventable complications from diabetes through healthy behavior change. I could give people hope along with tools to achieve the healthy goals they desire! This would be the most amazing thing that could come from losing my brothers, mom, and dad. They would be so proud of me! So, I'll ask you, those of you who are grieving, "What is the most amazing thing that could come from losing your loved one?"

One of the most amazing moments of the last several years was when I interviewed Kathrine Switzer for my podcast. If you don't know Kathrine, she was the first female to register and run the Boston Marathon. During the race, the race manager tried to physically remove her from the course. She went on to become a visionary and pioneer for women's marathon running and journalist and commentator. She's an extraordinary woman. I spent weeks preparing to talk with her. I read everything she'd written (if you haven't read *Marathon Woman*, you should, it's an incredible book) and a bunch of articles about her. I had met her over thirty years ago when I briefly worked for her in New York. I was so excited to connect with her again on my podcast. I was nervous but in a good way; this was going to be awesome!

I logged on and suddenly, there she was. The brilliant New Zealand morning sun streamed in through her window. We chatted for a few minutes and then jumped into recording the podcast. It was like catching up with an old friend. After it was over, I walked out of my recording space, and said to my husband, "That was so cool! I can't believe I just got to do that!" I had a huge smile on my face, and I was buzzing. I bounced around the house for the rest of the day. Why would I not want to allow myself to experience that kind of joy? Why not sit with the positive feelings like I have negative ones or the sad ones? Why would I want to downplay that amazing experience at all? It was one of the most fantastic things I'd ever done! I reveled in it, I savored it, and I still do.

About six weeks after the podcast episode dropped, Kathrine sent me an email. She told me she never listens to her interviews (and she's done thousands) but decided to listen to the podcast. She told me that she considered it one of the best and most important interviews she'd ever done. She complimented my interviewing skills because she had never shared so many personal details with anyone in an interview. You have to believe me when I tell you, I reveled in that email for a long time, too!! Better yet? I accepted the compliment and didn't dismiss it or minimize it. I owned it and it was a great feeling! What an amazing life I have.

I have a tendency to achieve things and then move on without taking the time to appreciate the accomplishment or even acknowledge that I reached a goal. Mom always told me to stop and relish those moments. The moments of accomplishment, of reaching what I thought were unattainable goals, and being present. She always wanted me to sit with them for a while and think about how I was feeling

My coach, Marcie, helped me do this. Every time we met, she asked me about my wins. It forced me to think about not only what my wins were but what I even consider a win. Trust me, my wins have changed considerably over time. I'm finally learning how to give my wins as much attention as my challenges. I like being present and congratulating myself now. It feels good. I enjoy being my own cheerleader and telling myself, *Good job, way to go!*

My favorite response to something I've done or experienced? *That was so cool!!*

Chapter Twenty

As a little girl, I carried the weight of the world on my shoulders. I had a lot of responsibilities that children probably shouldn't have had, but there I was. On one hand, it prepared me for a world where I would need those life skills. On the other hand, it was often overwhelming and paralyzing. I can't change anything about my past, but I realize that to move forward, I had to honor that little girl who felt invisible, who couldn't compete with the alcoholism, the hemophilia, and the accident that almost took my brother's life. Make no mistake, I always felt loved and never felt any of it was my fault. For that, I'm grateful. However, I realize now that my eating to self-soothe and comfort myself started at a young age and in order to start healing, I had to intentionally celebrate that little girl and let her know she did a good job. That she not only survived; she thrived.

If I could go back and tell her one thing, I would let her know that she was perfect just the way she was. That the world is waiting for her to make her own magic because, as I would find out, the magic lies within us. I'm proud of that little girl and I think she's proud of me.

Wherever you are in your journey, know that you are enough, more than enough. You are worthy, and when it's your time to shine, you will. No more hiding your light under a barrel. No more diminishing your light because others think it's too bright. As I've heard so many others say to those who were diminishing their value, their energy, "If my light is too bright, put on some sunglasses." Yes, this! Own your fabulousness in all its glory. Make an entrance! Be loud! Be YOU! Whoever that is, you be you. Don't let anyone else define you or tell you your worth. Don't relinquish that power to anyone. There is only one you and you are special! Believe it.

I believe that the only way to good health is through self-love. I believe the only way to transform ourselves is through self-love. In order to start my transformation process, I had to revisit a very injured little girl. I had to figure out what needed healing and start there. It wasn't about doing it to lose weight, it was to find out why I was overeating in the first place. It meant learning how to love myself unconditionally. I had to let go of the harsh language I used to talk about myself, the limiting thoughts, and the habits that derailed my success. I had to learn how to become my own number one fan. I finally figured out that treating myself with care, respect, and kindness was getting me a lot farther than shame, disappointment, and disgust. The world can be a cruel place, make sure you don't add to it by tearing yourself down and beating yourself up, too.

Change isn't easy but being honest with myself helped. I stepped out of denial and acknowledged my shortcomings, but I also shone the light on my gifts, strengths, and purpose. Only focusing on the negative wasn't going to help me heal. I had to celebrate the rest, too.

I urge you to keep going so you can see and embrace all that is good and beautiful and special about you. Don't just focus on the shortcomings or flaws, you have no idea how magnificent you already are.

I don't believe you can shame or hate yourself into good health. While I sure didn't start from a place of self-love, I actively worked on it, and it started to grow. I knew I couldn't tell myself I was disgusting, gross, or unworthy, and then expect myself to make healthy choices. While I couldn't be in denial about my health or the habits that got me here in the first place, bombarding myself with negative thoughts just derailed me. The world is mean enough. The hate messages hurled at those of us who are overweight or obese are plenty for a lifetime. I didn't need to pile it on from the inside, too.

It's hard to heal when you are constantly tearing yourself down. Just like a wound won't heal if you keep picking at it, I had to take a hard look at how I was treating myself. I had to start loving myself fully and unconditionally and in a way that supported the vision of my new life. I'm saying I had to love the innermost part of me, my soul, the essence of who I was. I had to start telling her how amazing she was no matter what the scale said. My family, friends, and coworkers would tell me how wonderful I was, but I never believed them. I finally asked myself, *Why not me?* Why can't I be wonderful and amazing and beautiful? They told me I was smart, but I dismissed that until I was halfway through my time at NYU. Even though I had gotten myself off academic probation earlier in my college career and even though I had gotten into NYU, I still did not see myself as intelligent. It finally dawned on me during the third or fourth semester that not only was I getting excellent grades on tests, but I was writing papers around complex concepts that were eliciting high praise from my professors. The feedback I was getting absolutely supported the reality that I was intelligent. I finally accepted that I was smart.

Whatever we tell ourselves, that is our reality. How we talk about ourselves, that's how we treat ourselves. That's the good news: We absolutely have the power to transform our lives, to achieve our goals and it starts by changing how we talk to ourselves. Once I started saying good things to myself, making healthier choices became much easier. I wish the process happened in a straight line, but it doesn't. It was usually two steps forward and one step back or even the other way around, but I kept going. Because I'm more conscious of how I talk to myself, I catch myself a lot faster and can course correct. I replaced negative self-talk with positive self-talk. I kept telling myself I was worthy, that I was worthy of putting in the extra effort and time it was taking to prepare meals, pack my lunches, and make sure there was healthy food in the house. I realized, and this was huge, that I was even worthy of inconveniencing others sometimes, if that's what it took. It's impossible to do any of that when deep down in your soul, you don't believe you deserve it.

One thing I keep working on is holding myself to such a high standard that I'm not allowing myself to make even the slightest mistake. I didn't realize I did this until recently. I'm incredibly forgiving when others screw up but me? I zero in on it, ruminate on it for days, and refuse to forgive myself for something others may not have even noticed. It just goes to show that even when I make progress in one area, there are other areas I still need to work on. I was emceeing a ceremony for work, and I blanked on the name of one of the physicians. Because of that, I didn't feel I could address the others by name either, so I introduced them as faculty of the program. I was mortified. It ruined the entire night for me, even though by all accounts it was a hugely successful evening. It bothered me that night and into the next day. I got to work and sent out an apology. No one responded. I, of course, thought it was because they were upset. It wasn't the case at all. They had no idea what I was talking about. I talked it through with some coworkers and no one could figure out what exactly it was that I was so upset about. They had attended and didn't notice anything wrong. I kept trying to convince them how badly I had screwed up. They were dumbfounded.

A friend of mine happened to call and I told her about it. She couldn't talk me off the ledge, either. No one could. It was getting ridiculous. Finally, after a full day of beating myself up, I sent a note off to Marcie. She sent me a response that finally calmed me down. This experience shone a very bright light on the work I still had to do. I had to find ways to stop this from happening in the future. I had figured out how to not beat myself up about overeating, but it just shifted to something else. My therapist has since given me a few tools to help me reframe these events and how to keep things in perspective. It's working.

Marcie once asked me: "How do you feed your spirit?" I thought it was a great question. I thought of it as another way of asking how I talk to myself. Is it a steady diet of hateful, nasty comments, or do I remind myself that I am a beautiful human being who is still learning and growing and evolving? Do I protect myself by putting myself in healthy environments or do I keep allowing myself to stay in dysfunctional circumstances that make me feel less than? We've all done it. Most of us for a very long time. Sooner or later, though, I hope you'll realize how truly special you are and that you deserve to love yourself and to be loved in a healthy, supportive way.

Throughout this journey, I have become more self-protective of my life and my inner circle. I firmly believe that if someone doesn't make my life a better place to be or enrich it in some way, then I either limit the time I spend with them or I don't interact with them at all. I realize that sometimes it's family who are toxic or unhealthy and that's unfortunate and painful, but we still need to take care of ourselves and if that means limiting interaction, so be it. Frankly, if I was making someone feel bad about themselves (and I hope that's never the case), they shouldn't hang out with me, either!

Therapy has been incredibly helpful for me even though I didn't start going to therapy to figure out why I ate so much or was self-soothing with food. Grief brought me to therapy. After Eric died, loved ones would check in with me asking if I was okay. I told them that I would know when it was time to get help. I was doing fine until I wasn't. I was really angry at everyone, at life. I was snapping at people at work and at home. After one particular overreaction at work, I knew I had to do something. I realized I wasn't doing ok.

I asked for some recommendations and found Heather. As angry as I was, I was in tears in minutes. I mean sobbing. As hard as it was to admit I needed help, it has made a world of difference. Trying to deal with Eric's death is what got me into therapy, but figuring the rest of it out is what's keeping me in therapy. I'm dealing with some of my childhood traumas that impacted my life, like my father's alcoholism. It was an important place to start but that wasn't all of it. We all have complicated lives and it's helpful to have someone help us unpack it. I'm finding that to be valuable and freeing.

At my first session, I was sitting on my therapist's couch having just shared the Cliff Notes version of my life: growing up in an alcoholic home, being a three-time cancer survivor, burying my entire family, being diagnosed diabetic, losing 110 pounds, and, finally, what specifically prompted me to seek help.

Heather looked at me and said, "That's a lot to deal with, and yet, you're still here. Where do you get your strength?"

I sat there for a minute. I was stumped. I had no idea how to answer that question. I said, "I don't know. I guess I don't know how else to be."

To myself, I thought, *What was the alternative except just getting through it? I didn't know what else I was supposed to do.* As a young girl, my mom depended on me. I was practically raising my little brother because she worked and was having to deal with Dad and Chris's hemophilia. I didn't think it was an option to not do that. Even in adulthood, I always just put one foot in front of the other and I showed up. I do what I have to do even when I'm not sure what that is.

So, where *did* I get my strength? How could I be so resilient? It was a nagging question that I didn't feel I had a good enough handle on and then, I finally figured it out. I realized that I was looking at it wrong; I was only looking inward for the answer. In this case, I needed to look outward, too. I needed to look around me. I realized it wasn't just about me; it was about my environment, my family, my friends, and even my ancestors. I finally understood. When I was going through the most difficult times in my life, I was being held. I was being held up by love both physically and emotionally. I never had to walk through any of these experiences alone. Ever. I always had someone there who supported me, who showed up to cook for me when I was sick, who was there when someone died, when I had to do the very things I thought I could not do. They held me up so I could lean into whatever it was that I had to do. Sometimes it was physically holding me up, sometimes it was through prayer, and sometimes it was by creating an environment so I could focus on my cancer or my loss and not have to worry about anything else.

Looking back, it's so clear. When I had cancer the first time, when I was living in New York, my mom and her sisters stayed with me. They cooked, they cleaned, they made me laugh. They held me when I was in pain, and they were then when I had my surgeries and treatments. When I had thyroid cancer the second time, my brother, Eric, came down to live with me, cook for me, and walk with me through treatments and scans. They were there when I was literally radioactive and unsteady when I finally received treatment. They held me close when I needed them to, and they always have. They always will. When I lost Eric, Ronn held me up and gave me space to grieve. There are still days when he has to hold me a little tighter.

I'm not saying I don't have any internal strength or that I'm not resilient, clearly, I am. However, I don't believe I could have gone through most of what I've dealt with without the support of others. I believe it even goes beyond those who are physically with me today. I believe those who have already passed are holding me in their love. I know Mom, Dad, Chris, and Eric are. I'm sure my grandparents and relatives who I held so dear and were such a huge part of my life are still holding me in the light.

My point is, for some reason, some of us think when we are going through something difficult, we should only look inward for strength and resilience. That reaching outward for support means we're weak. I finally realized that I found my strength from looking outward. I let my loved ones hold me close, which gave me the strength to do the hard work. To lean in and face whatever I was facing. I was never alone. I don't believe I could ever be that strong on my own. No one can. Let yourself be held. Let them hold you as you walk through difficult times. Don't be afraid; they won't let you fall.

When I look back over my entire life, which is what therapy often helps you do, I realize that even as a young girl, I was strong. I went through a lot, but I survived. As an adult, I've been through a lot, as well, and have survived. Actually, I have thrived in spite of it all, or maybe, because of it all.

Chapter Twenty-One

Throughout this journey of self-discovery, I've learned a few things. I learned I'm worth taking the extra time it takes to make sure I have what I need. I have no problem inconveniencing myself or going the extra mile for someone else, but for me? I'm not so quick to do that. I love helping other people. Always have. However, I never felt comfortable inconveniencing other people or asking them to pivot or even to wait a few minutes to support me. In essence, I was telling myself that I am not nearly as important as someone else is. That had to stop. I found that something as simple as taking the time to prepare the food I need to keep myself healthy is one very visible way I am taking care of myself. It communicates to them that I know I'm important, too. It also shows others how to take care of their own needs, too, and how not to always put ourselves last.

For a while, I'd had no problem staying within the two- to three-pound range I set for myself. Up a little? Adjust. I'd settled into a comfortable pattern, maybe even a little complacent. I knew what to eat and how to eat. I was moving more and intentionally trying to fit additional movement into my day. I had been in therapy for almost a year and was feeling pretty good. So good, in fact, that I stopped going. I rationalized that I was taking a break because we had moved to a new house an hour away. I needed time to adjust to my new commute and then I would be back. Five months later, I had yet to go back.

Little by little, things started building up and falling apart. It was subtle at first, almost unnoticeable. I started snacking more. Not a lot, just a little. I started to relax my portions. Not a lot, just a little. I started to move less. Then I became stressed about a couple of things, and then I got the flu, which meant a steroid shot. Steroids are wonderful drugs, but they can wreak havoc on your appetite and emotions. They sure did mine. I had a complete meltdown one weekend. I was questioning everything. My purpose. My value. My podcast. My book. Everything. I was in tears and Ronn was trying to figure out what was going on. Steroids can do that, for sure, but there was something else going on. I was up eight pounds. I felt so defeated. My main indicator light that something was wrong was flashing bright red!

Inherently, there's nothing wrong with having a meltdown but, obviously, something was wrong. Things had been building up and I hadn't noticed, or I ignored it. I needed to do something, but I wasn't sure what. For the record, if I go into meltdown mode, I embrace it. I go all in! I go straight to feeling like nothing I'm doing has value and that I'm useless. Yep, my inner bully starts to roar, and I listen to it and own it all. The problem is that it isn't true. None of it. But in that moment, I accept it all. I own it. After I ranted and raved for a while, I realized what was going on, what I needed to do. First, I needed to get some sleep. A good night's sleep often provides clarity, and it did for me once again. On Monday morning, I called my therapist and made an appointment. Throughout the week, I was starting to process everything and make sense of what was going on. There was a lot going on at work which was causing me to feel anxious. It wasn't the work itself; it was other dynamics. Things I couldn't control. Heather helped me put things back in perspective and helped me figure out what had triggered some of my reactions. As usual, I wasn't feeling heard, and I was getting dismissed. When my values are ignored, I feel it immediately. Talking it out helped me put labels on what was going on which helped me process. I felt infinitely better when I left her office.

I also happened to have a session with my Marcie that Friday. I told her what happened and what she helped me realize is that we all have foundations that we have to treat as sacred. When those get fractured or damaged, we must be committed to making sure we go back and get them back in place or everything else will crumble. That's what happened to me. I realized that I need to talk with someone to help process my life, my stressors, my sources of pain or anxiety. If I don't, I let it all build up until I can't handle it anymore, and then it impacts all aspects of my life: mental, emotional, physical, and spiritual. If I'm not actively and health-fully processing my emotions, I start to eat. I need to remember that self-soothing with food is what I do. It's my default behavior, so if I find myself overeating, something is wrong. I'm lucky it manifests in such an obvious way even if it takes me a while to recognize it. It prevents me from going too far down the rabbit hole. I can course correct earlier and, if I'm paying attention, learn some things about myself. I have to be open to that or what's the point of going through these experiences?

I realized my foundations are therapy, staying true to my values (being seen and heard are two major ones), and maintaining an honest relationship with myself. Denial and justifying my behavior are dangerous for me. For me to live a healthy life, I have to have all three legs of the stool in place which means I have to nurture and protect them. If these are in place, I can do more, love more, and live more. Without them, I falter and revert to old, unhealthy behaviors and thinking.

What I'm most proud of throughout this experience is that I was never embarrassed. I didn't apologize for being human. I genuinely wanted to figure out what was going on and if a meltdown helped me move forward, so be it. Ronn understood I was struggling and was as supportive as ever. He also understood that I would find my way through it eventually even if it wasn't pretty. Ronn always listens and does whatever he can do but we both realize, sometimes I need to talk to a professional. The best news was I never once considered giving in and just starting to eat. There's always a powerful pull to say, "What the hell, I screwed up, I might as well give up." That was a huge win for me.

What are your foundations? What must be in place for you to live your best life? What do you need to treat as sacred? What do you need to protect?

Someone once told me to own what's mine, but not what belongs to other people. As women, we tend to take on others' burdens and even apologize for things we didn't do. At least, I did. Revisiting my life has given me an opportunity to not only own what was mine but stop carrying everyone else's failures or responsibilities. I have enough on my plate, I don't need to carry everyone else's, too. Realizing this meant freedom and having the energy left for myself.

Since writing this book, I've realized I am a food addict. I'm not just addicted to sugar. I have always continued to overeat even when it caused negative consequences. I have always felt compelled to eat, sometimes it was out of my control, sometimes it wasn't. It's a challenge because we must eat and there are all sorts of ways to justify overeating. But just like my dad, I have slips. Some are small and some are profound, but the difference now is awareness. I know when I'm treading on thin ice, when I'm talking myself into eating more than I need, and when I'm justifying and in denial. When I feel myself slipping, I find it helpful to ask myself: *Is something bothering me? What am I avoiding? What am I trying not to feel?* None of us like discomfort, we all would like to feel good all the time or at least not feel so bad. But that's not how life works. Sometimes we're going to feel bad or sad or mad. I'm learning how to sit with that, realizing that it, too, will pass. I don't have to medicate with food. Sometimes I just have to be.

I'd been pretty successful maintaining my weight loss save for the previous uptick in my weight, but after Thanksgiving, I got the flu, and they gave me a steroid shot. Steroids make me hungry. I mean ravenous. While I surely didn't eat enough extra food to gain five pounds, the scale said otherwise. Two months later, it was still there. It would not budge. I was frustrated and tempted to give up and go back to my old habits. But I didn't, I focused on trying new strategies. This is part of the hard work that I knew was going to come with losing 110 pounds. It didn't make it any less frustrating, though.

I was talking with a new friend about my situation. I had met her at an international obesity and diabetes conference earlier in the year and she'd been a health coach for many years. I was curious to get her thoughts on my situation.

"It's driving me crazy," I told her, "No matter what I do, I can't get rid of the weight. I've gone back to basics, I'm watching everything I'm eating. I'm moving more. I increased my water. I don't know what else to do."

"It sounds like your body is holding on to the weight for some reason. Maybe it's time for you to stop fighting so hard."

I wasn't sure where she was going with this, so I just listened.

She asked, "Do you meditate?"

"Not really."

"It sounds like maybe you could benefit from just sitting quietly for a few minutes every morning. Just breathing. Accepting yourself and your body and then letting the excess weight go. Tell it while you appreciate it trying to protect you, but you're done with it now. It can leave. You have no use for it anymore."

Well, now. Interesting, I thought. I wasn't quite sure what I thought she'd say but that wasn't it. Obviously attacking it wasn't working. The scale was not budging. Maybe surrendering was the answer. Maybe doing some deep breathing would help. Maybe the harder I fought, the harder it was going to be to lose those extra pounds. Why not give it a try?

I never quite got the hang of meditation in the morning, but at night while saying my prayers, I decided to have a much more loving conversation with myself and that extra weight that wouldn't budge. I told it that I appreciated that it was trying to protect me, from what I didn't know, but apparently it was.

"Thank you, but it's time for it to go now. I had no more use for it. I was fine."

I kept tracking and doing all the same things I had been doing and a few weeks later, it was gone. Go, figure.

Time is a healer in its own way. I have some distance now from when I started Weight Watchers, reached my weight loss goal, and my brother's death. It's given me perspective. I think it's important to be honest with myself and looking back over the course of my life I have figured a few things out. First, I am a survivor. Wait—that's not quite true. I am a thriver. In spite of my challenges, in spite of the distractions and diversions and bad decisions, I am exactly where I am supposed to be. It has taken me a long time to accept that. I've spent most of my life believing that I needed to catch up, achieve more, make more money, and apologize for not being where my peers were. They say comparison steals joy and that's true. As Mom always said, "Don't compare your inside with other people's outsides." She was right, too; it's not a fair comparison. I lost every time.

Second, I'm stronger than I think I am. I've survived cancer, been diagnosed with diabetes, been morbidly obese, and buried my mom, dad, and both brothers. All of those experiences have contributed to how I live my life. Even with all the dysfunction, I was blessed with a family that loved me hard, and I deeply loved them back. We always had each other's backs. Even though there are days when I am deeply sad and miss them terribly, I still get great strength from them. Their impact on my life continues in very positive ways.

Third, I have always chased the light. No matter what was going on or what I was going through, I always found the light. Sometimes it took a while, but I never succumbed to the darkness. Looking back on my life, I can honestly say that I am proud of the woman I have become. While it wasn't always pretty, I always kept going. That is something to celebrate with intention. I also finally figured out that going through all I have gone through means something. I can't continue to dismiss it as though it was no big deal. It was all a big deal and just because I survived it, doesn't mean it wasn't. Lastly, I love generously. No matter what failings I have, and I have plenty, in the end, I still love deeply and that's all that matters. Isn't it?

Acknowledgments

Writing a book, any book, is hard. Writing a book based on your life is a whole other level of hard. You'd think it would be easy, after all, it's your life and you pretty much know all the facts, but it's not. At least it wasn't for me. For me writing a book that included the good, the bad, and the sometimes ugly required me to delve into some memories I had once thought were better left alone. I realized about halfway through that writing this book was healing me in ways I didn't know needed healing. It healed my soul through revisiting that little girl who thought she was invisible but found out she was anything but invisible. She found out she was strong and not just a survivor, but a thriver.

Everyone needs to get to know themselves, to find their voice. I just happened to meet the best version of myself a little later in life. To me, it doesn't really matter when you find your voice or your light, what matters is that you stay diligent and find it. I've found that the journey to true self-discovery begins when we start to peel away the layers of self-limiting thought and shame and find out what is important to us, what we value deep down in our being. What is important to us, not what we think is important or should be important, but what actually makes us light up inside or what makes us catch our breath. This is when we know we're on to something bigger than ourselves and, let me tell you, it's addictive.

All our lives are filled with ups and downs. I've experienced the highest of the highs and the lowest of the lows. What I've realized is that it was during the times I was most vulnerable that I learned the most about myself. When I was frustrated or scared or the times when I felt I was the weakest or most overwhelmed was when clarity came, if (and this is a big one), *if* I was open to making some changes. If we aren't open to changing what we are doing, how we are thinking, or what we believe about ourselves, then clarity will not come, and no transformation can occur. That's when my journey toward self-discovery really began. In taking this journey, I recaptured my purpose, my truth, my way forward, and my life. We all have a purpose, and no two paths are alike. Who would want to walk the same path as anyone else, anyway?

It was my goal that through sharing my story, you would see within yourself what is so very special, so unique, that only you possess it. I also hope you find all the strength and confidence you need to fully embrace who you are and finally believe in your own magic. It's there, trust me.

When it's the darkest, we have to find the light. Even if we can't see it right away, it's there, but we don't have to find it all on our own. There are always people in our lives, and not always the ones we think, who are there to hold us up when we feel we can't stand, to help us look inward (sometimes upward). They are always there to help us move through the dark. None of us can do this on our own. It doesn't matter how strong or weak you are, or how strong or weak you *think* you are, we need each other.

Life happens to all of us, but we always have choices. Traumatic events happen to everyone. You can either build mountains of them and let them define you, or you can lean in, walk through them the best you can, process the pain, gather the wisdom when it's time, and seek clarity. Then, you can let them transform you. You can choose to be bitter, or you can get better. You can be a passive participant in your life, or you can be the director. It's up to you. That's the good news.

If they ever made a movie about my life, it wouldn't be boring. I never seemed to take the safest path forward, nor the one that would bring me the most financial or emotional security. But it was the path I took and the fact that it brought me here, where I am today, was worth it. I have had to overcome my share of challenges, maybe more than my fair share, but I still see the good in people, in life, in the world. I still choose love, and I'll always choose the light over the dark.

I have to thank my editor, Amanda Edgar, PhD, and her team at Page and Podium Press, they made this process a little less daunting. I also want to thank Christi Pratt, who helped me get my manuscript ready to submit for review by lifting me up and showing me where the beauty lies within me. To those who encouraged me to write this and to keep going when I thought I couldn't do it, thank you. To Marcie and Heather who have been instrumental in guiding me in my journey. To my family who have gone before me: I love you and feel your presence daily. To Ronn, Branwyn, Joe, and the boys: you are my heart, and I am beyond grateful for having found you. I love you very much.

Gretchen

About the Author

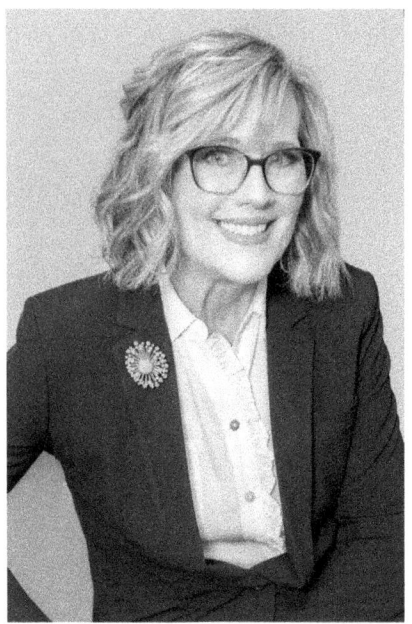

Gretchen Holmes, PhD is an experienced Graduate Medical Education professional and researcher, having published in top journals including Health Communication, Psycho-Oncology, and Injury Epidemiology. Her published research includes work in obesity management, rapport, provider-patient communication, health literacy, decision-making, and rural cancer health disparities. She has taught Behavior Change Theory at the Centers for Disease Control and Prevention, has served as a national-level patient advocate for the National Cancer Institute since 2002 and serves on the editorial board for the Journal of Patient Experience. She was named one of the Top 100 Successful Women to Know in 2022 by Gulf Coast Magazine. A three-time cancer survivor, Dr. Holmes is a motivational and keynote speaker and is the host of the podcast, "The Work in Between," that focuses on the daily behaviors and actions necessary to achieve our physical, emotional, mental, and spiritual health goals.

Dr. Holmes holds a Bachelor of Science and a Master of Arts in Communication from New York University and a PhD in Health Communication with a Graduate Certificate in Medical Behavioral Science from the University of Kentucky.

www.ingramcontent.com/pod-product-compliance
Lightning Source LLC
Chambersburg PA
CBHW051310120626
46547CB00015B/2172